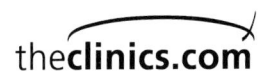

ORTHOPEDIC CLINICS OF NORTH AMERICA

Orthopedic Ancillary Services:
A Guide to Practice Management

GUEST EDITOR
Jack M. Bert, MD

January 2008 • Volume 39 • Number 1

SAUNDERS

An Imprint of Elsevier, Inc.
PHILADELPHIA   LONDON   TORONTO   MONTREAL   SYDNEY   TOKYO

W.B. SAUNDERS COMPANY
A Division of Elsevier Inc.

Elsevier Inc., 1600 John F. Kennedy Blvd., Suite 1800, Philadelphia, PA 19103-2899.

http://www.orthopedic.theclinics.com

ORTHOPEDIC CLINICS OF NORTH AMERICA
January 2008
Editor: Debora Dellapena

Volume 39, Number 1
ISSN 0030-5898
ISBN-10: 1-4160-5816-8
ISBN-13: 978-1-4160-5816-8

Copyright © 2008 by Elsevier Inc. All rights reserved. No part of this publication may be reproduced or transmitted in any form or by any means, electronic or mechanical, including photocopy, recording, or any information retrieval system, without written permission from the Publisher.

Single photocopies of single articles may be made for personal use as allowed by national copyright laws. Permission of the Publisher and payment of a fee is required for all other photocopying, including multiple or systematic copying, copying for advertising or promotional purposes, resale, and all forms of document delivery. Special rates are available for educational institutions that wish to make photocopies for non-profit educational classroom use. Permission may be sought directly from Elsevier's Global Rights Department in Oxford, UK: phone 215-239-3804 or +44 (0)1865 843830, fax +44 (0)1865 853333, email healthpermissions@elsevier.com. Requests may also be completed online via the Elsevier homepage (http://www.elsevier.com/permissions). In the USA, users may clear permissions and make payments through the Copyright Clearance Center, Inc., 222 Rosewood Drive, Danvers, MA 01923, USA; phone: (978) 750-8400, fax: (978) 750-4744, and in the UK through the copyright Licensing Agency Rapid Clearance Service (CLARCS), 90 Tottenham Court Road, London W1P 0LP, UK; phone (+44) 171 436 5931; fax: (+44) 171 436 3986. Other countries may have a local reprographic rights agency for payments.

The ideas and opinions expressed in *Orthopedic Clinics of North America* do not necessarily reflect those of the Publisher. The Publisher does not assume any responsibility for any injury and/or damage to persons or property arising out of or related to any use of the material contained in this periodical. The reader is advised to check the appropriate medical literature and the product information currently provided by the manufacturer of each drug to be administered to verify the dosage, the method and duration of administration, or contraindications. It is the responsibility of the treating physician or other health care professional, relying on independent experience and knowledge of the patient, to determine drug dosages and the best treatment for the patient. Mention of any product in this issue should not be construed as endorsement by the contributors, editors, or the Publisher of the product or manufacturers' claims.

Orthopedic Clinics of North America (ISSN 0030-5898) is published quarterly (For Post Office use only: Volume 38 issue 1 of 4) by Elsevier Inc., 360 Park Avenue South, New York, NY 10010-1710. Months of publication are January, April, July, and October. Business and Editorial Offices: 1600 John F. Kennedy Blvd., Suite 1800, Philadelphia, PA 19103-2899. Customer Service Office: 6277 Sea Harbor Drive, Orlando, FL 33887-4800. Periodicals postage paid at New York, NY and additional mailing offices. Subscription prices are $226.00 per year for (US individuals), $389.00 per year for (US institutions), $267.00 per year (Canadian individuals), $456.00 per year (Canadian institutions), $309.00 per year (international individuals), $456.00 per year (international institutions), $113.00 per year (US students), $154.00 per year (Canadian and international students). Foreign air speed delivery is included in all *Clinics* subscription prices. All prices are subject to change without notice. **POSTMASTER:** Send address changes to *Orthopedic Clinics of North America*, Elsevier Periodicals Customer Service, 6277 Sea Harbor Drive, Orlando, FL 32887-4800. **Customer Service: 1-800-654-2452 (US). From outside of the US, call 1-407-345-4000.** E-mail: elspcs@elsevier.com.

Reprints. For copies of 100 or more, of articles in this publication, please contact the Commercial Reprints Department, Elsevier Inc., 360 Park Avenue South, New York, New York 10010-1710. Tel. (212) 633-3813 Fax: (212) 462-1935 e-mail: reprints@elsevier.com.

Orthopedic Clinics of North America is covered in *Index Medicus, Cinahl, Excerpta Medica, and Cumulative Index to Nursing and Allied Health Literature.*

Printed in the United States of America.

ORTHOPEDIC ANCILLARY SERVICES: A GUIDE TO PRACTICE MANAGEMENT

GUEST EDITOR

JACK M. BERT, MD, Adjunct Clinical Professor, University of Minnesota School of Medicine, Summit Orthopedics, Ltd., St. Paul, Minnesota

CONTRIBUTORS

ANDREW J. BERT, BS, CPA, MST, Minneapolis, Minnesota

JACK M. BERT, MD, Adjunct Clinical Professor, University of Minnesota School of Medicine, Summit Orthopedics, Ltd., St. Paul, Minnesota

WILLIAM A. BOLESTA, MS, BOC, Board of Certification Orthotist; President, Orthotic Consulting Services, Hampstead, Maryland

KEN BROCKMAN, CPA, Summit Orthopedics, Ltd, Woodbury, Minnesota

DANIEL A. BUEHLER, AIA, Vice President, Facility Management and Construction Group, AmSurg, Nashville, Tennessee

ROBERT CIMASI, MHA, ASA, CBA, AVA, CM&AA, CMP, President, Health Capital Consultants, St. Louis, Missouri

PAUL DUXBURY, PT, ATC/R, Maplewood, Minnesota

DEBORAH GIANNINI, RN, CNOR, Director of Perioperative Services, Landmark Surgery Center, Saint Paul; Woodbury Ambulatory Surgery Center, Woodbury, Minnesota

DAVID M. GLASER, JD, Esq., Fredrikson & Byron, Minneapolis, Minnesota

TRENTON R. MATTISON, MHA, Regional Director, AmSurg, Dallas, Texas

DANA E. MAYBERRY, BS, Development Marketing Manager, AmSurg, Nashville, Tennessee

LOUIS F. McINTYRE, MD, Westchester Orthopedic Associates, White Plains, New York

WALTER O'NEILL, BS, R-PA, Orothopedic Imaging Partners, LLC, Verona, Wisconsin

JUDY POLASKY, Director of Medical Legal Services, Edina, Minnesota

STEPHANIE ROZMAN, Chief Executive Officer, Edina, Minnesota

VICTORIA L. RUDE, Esq., Chief Operating Officer, Edina, Minnesota

PAUL M. TORGERSON, JD, Dorsey & Whitney LLP, Minneapolis, Minnesota

ROBERT B. WEEKS, BS, MT, MA, Director of Marketing, Minnesota Occupational Health, St Paul, Minnesota

CONTENTS

Preface   xi
Jack M. Bert

Ancillary Services Available to the Orthopedic Surgeon   1
Jack M. Bert

> The delivery of high quality medical services is approaching a crisis situation in the United States. As physician reimbursements decline and overhead increases, orthopedic surgeons must seek additional sources of revenue to remain financially viable and control the quality of medical care that they deliver. The orthopedic surgeon group is well positioned to control its own service lines and deliver excellent patient care as a result. This article reviews the possibilities of multiple types of ancillary service lines available for the orthopedic group practice.

How to Perform a Feasibility Study and Market Analysis to Determine if an Ancillary Service Makes Sense   5
Ken Brockman

> A feasibility study, as the name implies, is a study of the viability of a business venture. The study is an analysis of the market potential of the new products or services to be offered and investigates the primary issues related to the new business. This article discusses the elements that are essential for a valid feasibility study.

Pros and Cons of the Ambulatory Surgery Center Joint Venture   11
Deborah Giannini

> If a physician group has determined that it has a realistic patient base to establish an ambulatory surgery center, it may be beneficial to consider a partner to share the costs and risks of this new joint venture. Joint ventures can be a benefit or liability in the establishment of an ambulatory surgery center. This article discusses the advantages and disadvantages of a hospital physician-group joint venture.

Developing an Orthopedic Ambulatory Surgery Center   17
Daniel A. Buehler, Trenton R. Mattison, and Dana E. Mayberry

> Although there are risks, the potential benefits should encourage one to consider developing an orthopedic ambulatory surgery center (OASC). Patients should appreciate the enhanced care they experience at a surgery center. The orthopedist can enjoy the benefits of increased income, time savings, and productivity provided by the surgery center. This article discusses the complex and time-consuming demands of developing

the OASC, and having it operate efficiently. It points out how experts can assist in developing and managing a highly efficient center, freeing the orthopedist to concentrate on performing surgery in an environment that is clinically, financially, and personally rewarding.

Financing and Cash Flow Management for the Medical Group Practice   27
Andrew J. Bert

> The expansion of a medical group practice and the addition of ancillary services require a substantial cash outlay. Obtaining proper financing to complete a successful expansion is a process that takes time, and there are critical steps that must be followed. The group's business objectives must be presented properly by developing a business plan detailing the practice and goals associated with the desired expansion. This article discusses some of the key elements that are essential in creating an overall effective business plan for the group medical practice.

Gain-Sharing with the Hospital: What is Possible in the Current Legal Environment   33
Paul M. Torgerson

> This article focuses on the idea of gain-sharing, defined as engagement between the hospitals and physician to create effective joint processes, common outcome measures, joint accountability, and a sharing of results. Gain-sharing is a logical approach to addressing fragmented care, cost containment, and improved clinical outcomes. In particular, this article focuses on contracts under which a hospital or institutional provider retains an independent clinic or physicians to tackle specific issues of service line performance.

The Physician-Owned Imaging Center   37
Walter O'Neill

> The advent of advanced imaging modalities in the past 20 years represents a paradigm shift as physicians seek new ways to offer earlier diagnosis and treatment and to augment practice service and revenues. A physician-owned, office-based imaging project has evolved from conventional X ray to more advanced imaging, which includes MRI, CT, and other digital imaging methods. Orthopedic practices need to do a thorough analysis to match the technology and type of unit to the patient volume and prospective payment for the services rendered. This analysis should include understanding the capability and limitations of the MRI or other imaging modality selected, staffing, siting, and teleradiology interpretations. This article elucidates this general trend in orthopedic imaging and examines practical aspects of the physician/practice-owned imaging center.

The Physician-Owned Physical Therapy Department   49
Paul Duxbury

> As the trend toward shrinking reimbursement for physician services continues, an internal physical therapy clinic providing high-quality care and a source of additional revenue presents an attractive opportunity. Internalization of physical therapy services within the clinic as either an off-site or on-site entity can assure patient access to the highest quality of rehabilitation services under the group's supervision and direction. It

will contribute positively to creating patient loyalty to and confidence in their physician and physical therapist. This article discusses the issues that are important to address in creating a physician-owned physical therapy department.

The Physician-Owned Occupational Health Department   55
Robert B. Weeks

This article provides a process to evaluate the likelihood of establishing a financially viable occupational medicine program (OMP), and discusses opportunities in which the occupational medicine clinic can partner with employers to help them to reduce the occurrence of work-related injuries and provide a safer work environment. Not all germane topics are discussed—employers must address safety and ergonomic issues within the workplace as well as those that a successful OMP is designed to address. However, the OMP should be a readily available resource for any of these issues. Common occupational challenges and opportunities also are examined.

The Physician-Owned Orthotic and Durable Medical Equipment Service   71
William A. Bolesta

In recent years, orthopedic practices have been forced to create internal ancillary profit centers to help compensate for escalating operating expenses. Increased professional liability premiums and health care costs, coupled with decreased reimbursements, have made the development of these ancillary centers a necessity. Practices that assess and incorporate sound business polices in developing the entity, monitor its progression, and strive to enhance the overall offerings within the division will derive the most profitability. By following a structured plan, practices can maximize revenue potential and improve patient satisfaction and outcomes. This article describes how to construct and follow such a plan.

Medical Opinions: The Physician-Owned Independent Medical Examination Company   81
Stephanie Rozman, Victoria L. Rude, and Judy Polasky

This article discusses the factors that contribute to the success of an independent medical examination company. It considers opportunity costs, the regulatory environment, the assessment of the competition and the customer base, and marketing principles. It also details the management expertise and the staff skill sets required for a successful venture.

Legal Issues Affecting Ancillaries and Orthopedic Practice   89
David M. Glaser

The federal and state governments have imposed significant regulations on health care generally and on ancillary services in particular. This article focuses on how state and federal laws shape the ability of an orthopedic physician to offer ancillary services, whether as an individual, through a group practice, or as part of a joint venture. It focuses on how the Stark law, the Medicare anti-kickback statute, state anti-kickback, fee-splitting provisions, certificate of need laws, and various Medicare billing and supervision requirements impact the provision of ancillary services. It also briefly discusses how physicians should prepare for and respond to government investigations.

The Attack on Ancillary Service Providers at the Federal and State Level   103
Robert Cimasi

> The health care delivery system in the United States has witnessed more dramatic changes during the last decade than it had since the passage of Medicare. The managed care revolution and changes in reimbursement for Medicare services have forced providers to look for more efficient ways to provide services as well as for additional sources of revenue- and margin-producing business. The move toward specialized inpatient and outpatient facilities, often owned by physicians, is a natural reaction to these significant changes. These developments have resulted a "turf war" between physicians and hospitals over who should control these revenues.

Making the Electronic Medical Record Work for the Orthopedic Surgeon   123
Louis F. McIntyre

> This article explores the current reasons why orthopedic surgeons might consider the adoption of an electronic medical record system in their practices today. The costs and benefits as well as the barriers to implementation are discussed.

Putting It All Together: The Efficient, Profitable Orthopedic Practice   133
Jack M. Bert

> In today's complex practice environment, the orthopedic surgeon is faced with multiple stressful practice decisions. To achieve a surgeon's personal practice goals of quality of care, quality of life, and improvement in quality of practice, the physician must commit himself or herself to a certain amount of restructuring of his or her practice. This article describes the elements necessary for successful restructuring.

Index   137

FORTHCOMING ISSUES

April 2008
> **Elbow Trauma**
> Scott P. Steinmann, MD,
> *Guest Editor*

July 2008
> **Patellofemoral Arthritis**
> Wayne Leadbetter, MD,
> *Guest Editor*

October 2008
> **Shoulder Trauma**
> George S. Athwal, MD, FRCSC,
> *Guest Editor*

RECENT ISSUES

October 2007
> **Scoliosis**
> Anthony A. Stans, MD,
> *Guest Editor*

July 2007
> **Minimally Invasive Spine Surgery**
> Dino Samartzis, DSc, MSc, Dip EBHC,
> Francis H. Shen, MD,
> D. Greg Anderson, MD,
> *Guest Editors*

April 2007
> **Wrist Trauma**
> Steven Papp, MD, MSc, FRCS(C),
> *Guest Editor*

The Clinics are now available online!

Access your subscription at:
http://www.theclinics.com

Preface

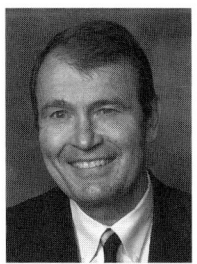

Jack M. Bert, MD
Guest Editor

The addition of ancillary services is necessary and critical to an orthopedic group practice's financial success, as well as its ability to control the patients quality of care. As reimbursements from clients continue to decline, the orthopedic group must develop alternative sources of revenue while remaining cognizant of the difficulties associated with doing so.

In the past year, as many as 31 states have proposed legislation aimed at preventing physicians from owning and controlling their own ancillary services. Powerful lobbying groups at federal and state levels have encouraged legislators to pass bills that would, in effect, force all surgical cases to be performed at non-physician–owned hospitals, restrict physician ownership of MRI units, and prevent physicians from owning physical therapy departments. If this happens at federal and state levels, a monopoly in the marketplace will occur, and healthcare costs will dramatically increase.

Only physicians possess the knowledge and capabilities to determine what is optimal care for any patient! By owning and controlling ancillary services, the physician determines who will care for his patient at every treatment level.

This issue of *Orthopedic Clinics* describes what ancillary services are available to the orthopedic surgeon, but, more importantly, it discusses how and when to determine if a specific ancillary service makes sense for the group practice. Feasibility studies and market analyses are critical aspects of determining if an ancillary service is appropriate for the group practice. The economics of developing an ambulatory surgery center, as well as whether to partner privately or with a hospital system, is discussed. Financing and managing cash flow for the orthopedic group and whether gain sharing is possible in light of the Stark regulations are other topics reviewed. Specific ancillaries, including MRI, physical therapy, occupational medical departments, durable medical supplies and physician–owned IME companies, are discussed in terms of the pros and cons associated with developing each service. The advantages and disadvantages of the electronic medical record and a discussion of the legal issues impacting ancillary services are thoroughly reviewed. The attack on physician ownership that is occurring at federal and state levels by those who wish to control healthcare delivery is discussed, and a summary of how to develop an efficient, profitable orthopedic practice is presented to conclude the issue.

Hopefully, these articles will help educate the orthopedist who is contemplating adding additional revenue sources to his practice on how to avoid the complications and pitfalls associated with developing these service lines in today's medical environment. It is my hope that we can maintain our private orthopedic surgical practices now and in the future and afford our patients the highest quality of care by controlling how care is delivered, as opposed to someone else telling us where, how, and by who it is delivered.

Jack M. Bert, MD
University of Minnesota School of Medicine
Summit Orthopedics, Ltd.
17 W. Exchange Street, Suite 307
St. Paul, MN 55120, USA

E-mail address: bertx001@tc.umn.edu

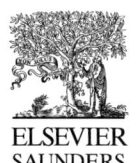

Ancillary Services Available to the Orthopedic Surgeon

Jack M. Bert, MD

Summit Orthopedics, Ltd., 17 W. Exchange Street, Suite 307, St. Paul, MN 55102, USA

The delivery of medical care services is approaching a crisis situation in the United States. As reimbursements decline and overhead increases, orthopedic surgeons must seek additional sources of revenue to remain financially viable. The orthopedic surgeon group is well positioned to manage its own service lines and obtain facility fees and other passive income as a result. This article reviews the possibilities of multiple sources of ancillary revenue for the orthopedic group practice.

The current climate

The delivery of medical care is the only business in which the customer tells the provider of a service what he will be paid without any recourse. Medicare, health maintenance organizations (HMOs), indemnity insurers, and all other payers including worker's compensation are seeking reductions in reimbursements to physicians as health care costs continue to escalate. As physician incomes decrease and overhead increases, physicians are seeking alternative but coincident sources of income by integrating ancillary services formerly controlled by hospitals and radiologists into their group practices. Unfortunately, this approach has resulted in the animosity of both the American Hospital Association and American College of Radiology, which have lobbied aggressively to remove specialty physician ownership of ancillary services. In 2004, legislation banning physician ownership and/or supporting or expanding certificate of need (CON) laws was introduced in more than 30 states (K. Bryant, personal communication, 2005).

This desire to obtain legislation banning physician ownership of ancillary services is a result of the dramatic increase in health care costs so that every provider (physician and hospital) wants a larger portion of the available health care dollar. Furthermore, the Center for Medicare and Medicaid Services (CMS) is planning a 29% decrease in physician fees by 2011 [1]. Thus, the desire to implement other revenue sources by physicians continues to increase.

Ways in which physicians can increase their revenue include the addition of ancillary services and businesses to their practices, increasing their local market share through growth and expansion, improving physician and office efficiency, improving payer contracts, hiring good management and decreasing office overhead, improving billing and collections, and, finally, maximizing coding reimbursements.

Orthopedic surgeons are one of the few subspecialties that are able to own and control multiple ancillary services to which that they can refer patients. In some states, however, the CON laws restrict ownership of certain ancillaries. Possibilities include in-house or freestanding ambulatory surgery centers (ASCs), MRI units, physical therapy departments with orthotics and braces, in-house durable medical equipment (DME), occupational medicine departments, independent medical examination companies, and in-office pharmacies. Some orthopedic groups offer retail sales of orthopedic or pharmaceutical equipment, have in-office pharmacies, and provide innovative therapies as well [2]. Gain-sharing arrangements with hospital systems, including hospital service management agreements, are becoming more commonplace as hospital systems realize the advantages of working collaboratively instead of competitively with group physicians (P. Torgerson, personal communication, 2005).

E-mail address: bertx001@tc.umn.edu

ASCs are perhaps the most common subspecialty ancillaries owned and operated by orthopedic surgeons in today's marketplace.

The in-office surgery center

The in-office surgery center or ASC has multiple advantages for the physician as well as for the patient. It allows more physician control of daily activities and hence improved productivity and revenue enhancement. Furthermore it provides better patient care. A recent study by the Office of Inspector General showed that 98% of Medicare patients were satisfied with their ASC experience, and 91% overall preferred the ASC to the hospital [3]. From the patient's perspective, in addition to greater satisfaction, the total operating room episode of care is shorter (average time in an ASC is 2.5 hours, compared with 4.5 hours for the same outpatient procedure). The infection rate is much less (0.15% compared with 4.0% for the same procedure in hospital), and the overall cost for the patients and the payers is lower [2].

The number of surgical cases treated in ASCs continues to increase and is expected to reach 50 million nationwide by 2007 (S. Iqbal, personal communication, 2005). The most profitable ASC cases, as evidenced by the outpatient surgery developer's survey, are orthopedics, hand surgery cases, podiatry, pain management, and ear, nose, and throat cases [4]. The first four of these specialties can be captured easily in an orthopedic ASC. Unfortunately, CON laws are a significant problem in more than 50% of the states at this time, and the National Hospital Association wishes to have CON laws present in all states because of hospitals' fear of competition for outpatient surgical cases. Further discussion of this problem and strategies to deal with this threat are discussed elsewhere in this issue. If physicians are able to lobby successfully in their respective states for maintaining ownership of their own surgery centers, the CMS will begin changing the way in which ASCs are reimbursed, which will help improve the revenues for orthopedic-focused ASCs. The ambulatory procedure code formula will be replaced by a reimbursement system that will be approximately 67% of the hospital outpatient payment rate mandated by HR 4042, the ASC Payment Modernization Act. Hopefully, dependent upon if the case is "device-intensive," most of the implant costs will be reimbursed.

It is critical to perform payer and market analyses when considering incorporating an ASC into the group practice. The "field of dreams" myth may not be realized (if you build it, they may not necessarily come) if preconstruction analysis is complete or appropriate. In addition to a thorough market and payer analysis, a political analysis also must be performed to avoid significant resistance to development of the ASC. The group's existing managed care relationships may have restrictive covenants as to where patients can have surgery. The group must analyze payer relationships before construction. Furthermore, if the payer has its own ASC or is affiliated economically with a hospital, the payer can avoid certifying the facility for reimbursement purposes. Also, the competing hospital or HMO can avoid credentialing its surgeons.

Two other articles in this issue provide additional guidance regarding the appropriate methods necessary to proceed in a stepwise fashion in the successful development of a physician-owned surgery center. It is crucial for the orthopedic group to prepare objective data before proceeding with the development of this project. It is important to choose high-quality, efficient surgeon investors who will perform profitable cases at the facility.

Determining financing needs and whether to chose a private partner or hospital system as a joint-venture partner is discussed elsewhere in this issue. The physician group should have equal or majority ownership of the ASC. The author of this article believes that management by the physician owners is mandatory. The ASC staff will be much more responsive to physician management than to hospital or corporate management.

Finally, a large practice with a high volume of outpatient cases that are "portable" (meaning that they can be taken to the ASC without restricted reimbursement) is imperative to ensure profitability. Obviously, a larger group practice can generate higher throughput (volume of cases performed in an ancillary service) than a smaller practice. A fixed overhead expense, such as rent, and variable overhead expense, such as the materials expense based upon case volume, is associated with each ancillary service. It is important to determine the volume of cases that realistically can be performed at the ASC before making a decision to proceed. Nursing staff should have excellent interpersonal skills to perpetuate an enjoyable, happy environment. This atmosphere will affect surgeon and patient satisfaction scores dramatically.

ASCs and in-office surgery centers are non-designated health care services and therefore are not governed by the Stark Law and Safe Harbor regulations. The remaining ancillary services discussed in this issue, however, are considered designated health care services and are regulated by Stark Law and Safe Harbor Laws that are discussed in detail later.

In-office MRI units

The in-office MRI unit can be extremely beneficial to the orthopedic group practice. It allows dramatic efficiencies in scheduling as well as the ability to choose who reads the scan. Determining which patients are "portable" is critical to determine if revenue streams will result in profitability. As with any ancillary service, market and payer analyses must be performed before proceeding with purchasing an MRI unit. These analyses and the process of determining which unit is appropriate for the group are discussed elsewhere in this issue.

The American College of Radiology is attempting to disallow the certification of extremity scanners. Furthermore, it is attempting to petition Medicare to disallow facility fee reimbursements for noncertified scanners. In addition, it has attempted (and fortunately has failed) in several states to allow physician ownership of MRIs only if the physician has completed a radiology residency and is board certified.

Physical therapy services

Physical therapy can be a significant profit center for the ASC. It is an excellent source of referrals for orthotics and braces. If the physical therapist has his/her own provider number, it is unnecessary to have a physician on site for patient care and treatment. A thorough payer and market analysis and an objective volume estimate should be performed before considering the addition of this ancillary service to the orthopedic group practice. A thorough discussion of how to develop a physician-owned physical therapy department is presented later in this issue.

Occupational health services

Worker's compensation clinics can be a significant source of revenue to the orthopedic group practice. To be successful, however, this ancillary service requires a completely separate department with a significant number of business referrals. A study published in 2001 estimated that employers spend more than $120 billion on work-related injuries each year in the United States (T. Thurman, personal communication, 2001). A significant amount of ancillary revenue generated by the worker's compensation clinic can be referred to the orthopedic group practice. This issue is discussed thoroughly in a separate article.

An analysis of the employer market within a 20-minute drive of the delivery site is mandatory, and it may make sense to develop a totally separate site for the occupational medicine department rather than creating a separate clinic site within one of the group's offices.

Independent medical examination companies

It is estimated that more than 80 million referrals for IMEs (independent medical examinations) are made each year, representing an estimated $180 billion spent for these medical opinions. If the orthopedic group sets up an independent medical examination company using only practicing orthopedists and other subspecialists to generate group revenue, the physician can supplement his practice revenue significantly as clinical reimbursements continue to decrease. This ancillary service requires a separate excellent manager who is skilled in dealing with defense insurers and both plaintiff and defense attorneys who control this market. The ability to generate this type of revenue varies among states and depends on the reimbursement for both worker's compensation and personal injury. A thorough review of this topic is presented elsewhere in this issue.

In-office durable medical equipment

DME is often a "loss leader" for some orthopedic practices because of the tendency to bundle all DME into global fees. It is critical to understand what necessitates reimbursement for DME. Knowing the requirements for precertification, which items can be billed separately to the patient, and which DMEs are reimbursable by each payer are only a few of the important requirements for realizing a positive cash flow with these supplies. This concept is discussed in a separate article in this issue.

Group size

Increasing group size is a major advantage when attempting to develop ancillary services for the orthopedic group practice. As noted, maximizing profits from ancillary services requires significant throughput because of the significant fixed overhead associated with each ancillary service. Furthermore, a larger group has the ability to control the marketplace as much as possible with multiple locations and referral sources so that the payers are forced to use the group. Increasing market share and diversity allows the group to avoid single-payer preferences so that the group cannot be "held hostage" for reimbursement by a single payer. A secondary benefit of greater group size is the ability to provide services in multiple locations, thus improving patient convenience and satisfaction. Often, if the group is large enough and has sufficient market share, ancillary services such as MRIs and physical therapy can be duplicated at various locations. Occasionally, economies of scale can decrease costs and increase revenue. Multiple locations speed up growth in a mature marketplace. Furthermore, a group's negotiating ability improves dramatically with greater market share.

Unfortunately, physicians have a difficult time with mergers because of an innate resistance to change, fear of a different group "culture," and perceived loss of control. A solution to this problem is to form an umbrella corporation (UC) with separate divisions and multiple satellite locations. The UC is the parent company and is the contracting entity. It is comprised of board members from each group. The multiple groups are managed locally and are divisions of the UC. The UC must have a common provider number and at least a common pension plan to be considered a merged entity by the payers. The practice must consist of a "single legal entity," and at least 75% of patient care services provided by group members must be provided through the group and billed under a number assigned to the group. The group must pass the "unified business test" with a centralized decision-making body, consolidated billing, accounting, and financial stateaments, and centralized utilization review (D. Glaser, personal communication, 2003). The benefits of a UC are that it avoids "bigness" within each division, allows some economies of scale for purchasing and some common office functions, allows a wider geographic range, makes mergers much easier, and is a single contracting entity. Furthermore, it improves the group's ability to make multiple ancillary services tremendously profitable by increased patient volumes that offset fixed overhead.

Unfortunately, physician mergers are not common for several reasons. Physician personalities tend to hinder the group's ability to make appropriate business decisions: physicians tend to feel threatened by their physician competitors and react emotionally instead of using sound business practices to determine if a merger makes sense. In the general business community, mergers tend to occur so that larger groups or corporations can exert some control over the marketplace. The payers would rather have the orthopedic community remain fragmented so that larger groups do not increase their market share and then attempt to negotiate for higher reimbursements from a position of strength. Orthopedic colleagues in a community should not be each other's enemies. The government (CMS), insurers, HMOs, and in most instances the hospitals are continuously attempting to control and reduce reimbursements so that they capture more of the health care dollars than the orthopedist. The legislative process in each state continues to be manipulated by lobbyists attempting to propose bills to eliminate physician ownership of ancillary services.

Summary

The hallmark of a successful medical group is the ability to adapt constantly to the ever-changing health care delivery system (I. Harrison, personal communication, 2003). Wherever possible, it is important to integrate services and related businesses into the orthopedic practice to improve efficiency and patient care and, as a result, to enhance revenues. Because the physician group controls and manages the ancillary service, it can hire the best caregivers possible to achieve the best possible patient care and treatment. Finally, the orthopedist must pay attention to the political landscape in the community and at a state level. A lobbyist to monitor impending legislative efforts before they are enacted into law may be needed and can be shared jointly with several other groups that have the same goals.

Understanding the need to incorporate ancillary services into the orthopedic group practice may determine the group's economic survival and quality of care that they deliver. The remainder of this issue discusses how to integrate ancillary services into the orthopedic group's practice successfully and, more importantly, what one needs to know before beginning this endeavor.

References

[1] Moore B. Physician reimbursement. Physician Practice 2006;(1):5–8.
[2] Bert J. Ancillary services available to the orthopedic surgeon. Sports Med Arthrosc 2004;12(4):254–7.
[3] Daniels B. Ambulatory surgery centers. Outpatient Surgery 2006;(1):12–8.
[4] Iqbal S. Outpatient surgery. Developer Survey 2004;(1):7–11.

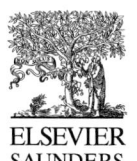

How to Perform a Feasibility Study and Market Analysis to Determine if an Ancillary Service Makes Sense

Ken Brockman, CPA

Summit Orthopedics, Ltd, 1860 Wooddale Drive, Suite 100, Woodbury, MN 55125, USA

A feasibility study, as the name implies, is a study of the viability of a business venture. The study is an analysis of the market potential of the new products or services to be offered. It is an investigation of the primary issues related to the new business.

The purpose of the feasibility study is simple. It decides whether to proceed with the proposed new business venture. Additionally, a thorough investigation will identify make-or-break issues that could prevent the venture from being successful. Determining early on that a business venture will fail saves time and money. Finally, the feasibility study provides the framework for a well-designed business plan.

A feasibility study must start with a clearly defined scope to provide focus to the investigation. Overly broad parameters on the scope have a negative effect on the results and conclusions of the study. The decision to conduct a feasibility study usually occurs after a number of ideas and alternatives have been presented. Defining the scope eliminates scenarios that do not make sense and, more importantly, identifies those scenarios that seem to have the potential for success.

The basic premise of a feasibility study is to determine the potential for success of a proposed business venture. As important as defining the scope is defining the anticipated end result, which is the successful ancillary service. A successful ancillary service is one that achieves the goals envisioned by the owners. Typically those goals include the ancillary service generating profits and cash flow sufficient to achieve a return on investment to the owners in proportion to their risk. In the field of health care, however, providing patients better access to high-quality, cost-effective medical products and services is as equally important in determining success of the ancillary service. High-quality health care must be provided for a new ancillary service to be viable long term.

It is important to highlight the distinction between a feasibility study and a business plan. A feasibility study determines if the business idea is viable and sound. It provides an investigative function. A business plan is the proposal to take the viable concept to reality. The business plan provides the planning function. It is compiled after the feasibility study is done, with the feasibility study being the basis for the business plan. The feasibility study may investigate several different scenarios, but the business plan focuses on the one best alternative based on the results and conclusions of the feasibility study. The business plan expands on the information contained in the feasibility study with a full analysis of the competition, the market, and several years of financial projections.

There are three components of a feasibility study: technical and organizational feasibility, market feasibility, and financial feasibility. Within each area, the specific constraints should be listed, risks weighed, and potential alternatives recommended.

The assessment of technical and organizational feasibility addresses and examines the key organizational and technology issues. Organizational issues include organizational structure, governance, management, and staffing. Technology

E-mail address: kbrockman@summitortho.com

issues focus on the availability, needs, and costs of technology as it impacts the new ancillary service.

Assessment of market feasibility concentrates on the market demand for the new products or services and on the current competition in the market. It determines whether the group can establish a market niche to compete effectively with others in the market. If the group cannot obtain sufficient market demand for its products or services, the new venture will not be feasible.

Financial feasibility is investigated after it is determined that the venture is market, technically, and organizationally feasible. Financial feasibility entails analysis of start-up costs, operating costs, revenue projections, and financing requirements. Financial projections should be completed with best- and worse-case scenarios.

Organizational feasibility as it relates to organizational structure and governance is a critical component of any health care ancillary service, given the numerous federal and state regulations with which one must comply. This article focuses on market and financial feasibility.

Market feasibility focuses on whether there is sufficient demand for the group's proposed products or services. Therefore it is essential to understand the current market. Understanding the market first involves an analysis of the competition, determining the number of other competitors in the geographic area providing the same or similar products or services. For example, if the group is contemplating a new physical therapy service or MRI scanner, the group needs to know the location and capabilities of other physical therapy clinics or MRI scanners that are available to patients. One should make certain to review all the potential capabilities of the new ancillary service. There may be a competitor in the market, but by providing better access for the patient (eg, through offering evening appointments or a more convenient location) the group may find a market niche that will make the ancillary service successful.

Equally important in the market analysis is understanding the current relationship that is in place within the practice and/or physicians and the facilities to which they refer patients. One should investigate the reason physicians use the current facilities or services. Does patient access, proximity to the clinic, or the quality of the MRI radiology reading dictate the MRI scanner to which the physician refers patients? Does block time scheduling, location, or turnaround time determine the outpatient center at which the physician performs a surgical case? Understanding these reasons is important if the group desires to redirect those referrals to an in-house ancillary.

Health system contracting also is an important factor in the market analysis. For example, a large percentage of the patient population in the Minneapolis/St. Paul metropolitan area is contracted by a few health care systems. Patients must be directed to providers or facilities affiliated or contracted with these health care systems. Such contracts are key factors in determining which patients can access in-house ancillary services.

Market feasibility, as stated, is a measure of demand for the proposed product or service. Demand equals volume of patients. Thus the most significant analysis to determine market feasibility is a volume analysis. How the group gathers the data for the volume analysis depends largely on which ancillary service the practice is considering. If the practice is considering an ambulatory surgery center (ASC), gathering the data is fairly straightforward, because the information is contained in the practice's billing system.

A report must be generated from the practice's billing system indicating the total number of outpatient cases performed by each physician in the previous 12 months. If the practice has more than one practice location, the report also must indicate the location at which the outpatient cases were performed. The "portability" of the patient cases from a geographic perspective must be factored into the volume analysis. The report also must indicate the Current Procedural Terminology (CPT) code for the cases performed. It is important to note the total number of outpatient cases performed, not the total number of CPT codes billed. Many of the surgical cases performed are billed with multiple CPT codes, depending on the type of procedure performed. Merely counting the CPT codes exaggerates the number of outpatient cases completed. Reviewing the physicians' surgery schedules will help verify the validity of the reported case volumes.

Gathering volume data for external referrals that the practice does not bill may prove difficult and time consuming. If the practice is considering an MRI scanner or a physical therapy clinic, and the practice does not track external referrals within the practice management system, it will be necessary to establish a specific system to quantitate those referrals. The tracking system may be either manual or integrated through the office practice management system. It will be necessary to quantify those referrals for at least a 3- to 6-month timeframe. When creating a template for tracking the external referrals, one should ensure that all the necessary data elements are gathered. It will become frustrating if the external referral data are gathered for 6 months only to discover that they are unusable because management failed to collect all the elements necessary to make a decision. Which data elements are gathered will depend on the capabilities of the proposed ancillary service. At a minimum, the group will need to record the type of procedure or product ordered, the requesting physician, and the payer. It may be necessary to collect other data elements, however. For example, if the practice is considering an extremity MRI scanner that has limitations as to where the scan can be performed, the size of the patient and type of scan that can be performed become crucial elements in performing volume estimates.

Developing consistent physician protocols also can assist in collecting data on potential volume for a proposed ancillary service. Establishing presurgical protocols for each of the physicians in the practice can be instrumental in determining if enough volume is present to include cold therapy or continuous passive motion units in a durable medical equipment (DME) ancillary service.

More critical than gathering the volume data is analyzing it properly. After the volume reports have been generated from the practice management system and external referrals have been tracked for at least 3 months, it will be important to evaluate the data to determine which patients or procedures are "portable." Portable patients or procedures are ones that can be redirected to an in-office ancillary.

A number of items must be taken into account to assess which patients or procedures are portable. First, it is important to understand fully the capabilities of the proposed ancillary service. If the group has decided to install an extremity MRI scanner, the group must review the volume data that have been collected to determine which scans can be performed with the newly proposed scanner. With an extremity MRI unit, the group may need to exclude cervical, lumbar spine, and pelvic scans. These data also may help determine whether a full-body or extremity scanner may be more feasible. Will the new physical therapy clinic have hand therapy? If not, any hand therapy referrals must be excluded from the physical therapy external referral data.

Second, one must understand regulatory limits on the new proposed services or products. Most of these limits will center on the Medicare guidelines; however, there also may be state regulations. For example, when analyzing the volume data for the new proposed ASC, one should note which ASC procedures are not approved by Medicare. Similarly, many DME products, such as continuous passive motion units and cold therapy, are not reimbursed by Medicare. These products and services must be excluded from payer volume estimates before determining whether the proposed ancillary service is feasible.

Third, the group must understand the health systems in the marketplace and how they will impact the referrals to the proposed, ancillary service. Larger, more coordinated health systems will already have many of their own ancillary services available to their members and will direct patients to those services. For example, health systems with physical therapy clinics typically restrict members to their clinics. It will be difficult to redirect those patients to the group's ancillary services. Even though it may be possible to redirect those patients to the group's physical therapy clinic and receive reimbursement from the payer, doing so may jeopardize referrals from primary care physicians employed by that health care system.

Finally, an analysis of the volumes by payer will be necessary to identify which procedures or patients can be redirected to the group's ancillary services. One should sort out the volume data by payer. The volume of each payer should be calculated as a percentage of the total, making certain to include all payers including workers' compensation, Medicare, Medicaid, and all major private payers, including managed care companies.

Analyzing the volumes by payer will entail two components. The first is determining whether the group will be able to obtain a contract with that payer for the new ancillary service. Some ancillary services will fall under the existing professional services contract, but others may require the group to obtain a new contract. Some insurance companies have closed networks on certain services, making it extremely difficult to obtain a contract. Insurance companies typically have credentialing and/or accreditation requirements. The payor may require an ASC to be accredited by Medicare or the Accreditation Association for Ambulatory Health Care. Certain payers require accreditation for MRI scanners. If the group is unable to or does not realistically foresee receiving a contract with a certain payer, these volumes must be excluded from the volume analysis. Second, even though a contract can be obtained for a payer, certain services or products may not be reimbursed at a level that makes these services or products financially viable. This situation is more common with an ASC or DME ancillary service: the cost of performing certain surgical procedures or dispensing certain DME products may be greater than the reimbursement from the payer. The group must exclude those services and products, as well, from the volume analysis.

The volume analysis provides the framework for the financial feasibility of the ancillary service. Based on the analysis described earlier, the care volumes should exclude services that the ancillary service will be incapable of performing, services limited by Federal or state regulations, by health system requirements, and by payers. The remaining volume is the "portable" volume, which often is 15% to 40% of the total volume of possible cases.

One other important factor in the market analysis is the legislative and regulatory outlook. A significant amount of state and federal legislation currently is being introduced that will impact physician-owned ancillary services. Anyone contemplating a new ancillary service must be aware of the current regulation affecting that ancillary and of any proposed legislation that could have a negative effect on that ancillary.

The final component of the feasibility study is determining financial feasibility of the newly proposed ancillary service. The assessment of financial feasibility includes an analysis of the start-up costs, operating costs, revenue projections, and financing requirements.

Start-up costs are the costs incurred in starting up a new business. They include capital goods such as facilities, equipment, and inventories and legal costs to establish the organizational structure. It will be necessary to estimate the initial start-up costs and also the capital needs required until revenues are at full capacity. Facility costs include projecting the design and buildout costs of the new facility space. If it is anticipated that land and building will need to be purchased for the new ancillary service, one must be certain to distinguish between the financial feasibility of owning the land and building and the feasibility costs of the new ancillary service.

It will be necessary to identify and assess the financing requirements. Will the funding come from equity or credit sources or a combination of both? If funding is from equity sources, a capital call structure must be projected. Funding from credit sources requires an assessment of the expected financing needs, including timing of loan advances, interest rates, terms, conditions, and covenants.

The results from the volume analysis of the market feasibility are the basis of the revenue projections. The projected reimbursement from each payor group must be estimated for all high-volume services or products. Projecting the reimbursement for the governmental payors will be fairly straightforward. Medicare, Medicaid, and workers' compensation have published reimbursement guidelines. Private payer reimbursement may be more difficult to determine; many, but not all, follow Medicare's schedules. An important distinction must be noted between the pricing or fee schedule for the various services and products and the contracted reimbursement from the payers. The revenue projections must incorporate the actual contracted reimbursement from the payer, not the billed charge that is submitted.

Finally, the operating costs must be projected. Operating costs are the ongoing costs, such as employee salaries and benefits, occupancy costs, and administrative costs, incurred in the everyday operation of the business. The operating costs should be divided between fixed and variable costs. Fixed costs are costs that do not vary based on the volume of services rendered, such as rent; variable costs, such as the cost of medical supplies, do vary with volume of services rendered.

The financial projections should include a break-even analysis. This analysis determines what volume of services or product sales must be achieved to cover the operating costs. Depending on the ancillary service, achieving break-even status may take from 6 months to a year. Thus, it is critical to ensure that the start-up period (the period before break-even is achieved) is funded properly.

The financial projections should be exhaustive and must include both best-case and worst-case scenarios. The group should benchmark the projections using published industry data. The Medical Group Management Association and the American Medical Group Association compile annual financial survey data. The group must prepare a projection of cash flow necessary for the start-up period. A full set of financial statements including the income statement, balance sheet, and statement of cash flows should be projected for a 3- to 5-year timeframe. The group must document fully the assumptions used in preparing the financial statements.

The final step in the feasibility study is a compilation of the results and conclusions. One should outline the various scenarios investigated, noting the implications of the findings and including the strengths and weaknesses of each. The results should help the group weigh the risks versus the rewards of setting up the proposed ancillary service. The feasibility study is designed to answer the question, "Should the group proceed with this business venture?" The answer is not always in the affirmative, so the group should be prepared for a negative conclusion. The final result will be either positive or negative, and the feasibility study is the major source of information when making the decision.

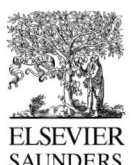

Pros and Cons of the Ambulatory Surgery Center Joint Venture

Deborah Giannini, RN, CNOR[a,b,*]

[a]Landmark Surgery Center, 17 West Exchange Street, Suite 310, Saint Paul, MN 55102, USA
[b]Woodbury Ambulatory Surgery Center, 8675 Valley Creek Road, Suite 300, Woodbury, MN 55125, USA

If a physician group has determined that it has a realistic patient base to establish an ambulatory surgery center (ASC), it may be beneficial to consider a partner to share the costs and risks of this new joint venture. Joint ventures can be a benefit or liability in the establishment of an ASC. This article discusses the advantages and disadvantages of a hospital physician-group joint venture.

There are several different types of joint venture partners. The group can partner with a nonsurgical physician practice, a multispecialty physician practice, a health maintenance organization (HMO), a hospital system, or an ASC specialty corporation. Hospital partnership and non-health care business investors (corporate-partnered) are the most common types of partnership.

Some of the advantages of a joint venture arrangement include: having the physician partner as the manager, participating in a shared investment and thus sharing its inherent financial risk, having an increased referral base if the hospital or HMO system controls family physician referral, and creating the possibility of increased efficiency and productivy. The disadvantages include sharing the profits generated by the surgeons, dramatic differences in management styles, and possibly having a partner with a conflicting vision for the joint venture.

* Woodbury Ambulatory Surgery Center, 8675 Valley Creek Road, Suite 300, Woodbury, MN 55125.
 E-mail address: dgiannini@summitortho.com

Pros of the ASC joint venture

Developing patient referral patterns

A significant advantage in partnering with a large health care entity is the ability to capture patient referral patterns for the new joint venture. Large health care groups may have many physician specialties within their work force. Family Practice and Internal Medicine areas are a prime source for surgical patient referrals. Marketing the group's availability to see a subspecialist may increase the revenue for the ASC joint venture. This is an opportunity for the physician group and hospital owner to increase patient volume, and thus revenue, by collecting a facility fee for each procedure performed at the center.

For the hospital partner, the opportunity exists to capture 50% of the facility fee by encouraging and monitoring their referring physicians to direct patient referrals to the new joint venture.

Reasons to direct the referral pattern to the new joint venture include;

1. Increased physician and patient satisfaction for receiving high quality, cost-effective care.
2. Efficiency, resulting in faster turn-over time than in an inpatient setting. Hospital operating room turn-over times average 20 to 40 minutes in-between procedures, whereas in an ambulatory surgery center setting, the turn-over time average is 7 to15 minutes, or even less depending on the procedure.
3. Ability to manage and thus provide direct input into the care and needs of the patient.
4. Potential for differential or tier placement ratings by various payers for providing high quality, cost-effective care.

5. Financial incentive for earning a profit from a well managed facility in which each partner has an ownership interest.

Potential for protection against legislation restricting ASC practice and development

At the state and federal levels, new legislation is being introduced every year to restrict or prohibit the future expansion of free standing ambulatory surgery centers. (Access Federated Ambulatory Surgery Association at www.fasa.org and click on the state updates to see what is being introduced in your area.)

Having a hospital partner in a joint venture has the potential to help curb these initiatives when the hospital partners are 50% owners of the venture. It would not be in the best interest of either owner to support legislation that would increase the cost of the center or place the center in jeopardy of trying to comply with new legislation. The greater the opposition to any legislation meant to restrict or prohibit the ability of the surgery center to operate or expand, the better off the ASC industry will be.

Physician owner as manager of the ASC

It is the belief of the ASC industry that physician owners are the best individuals to manage an ASC. It is felt that physician owners improve the quality of care for the patient. That is why it is crucial that once the group has decided on its partner, the management agreement should mandate that the physician partner will be the managing partner.

The physician partners have the expertise in developing and nurturing a more efficient, patient-centered model for the delivery of surgical services. The physician partner should seek clinical staff who are specially-trained, experienced, and highly skilled. The physician partner needs an ASC that is tailored to their specialty and operating style. The group will want to schedule procedures more conveniently for patients and themselves.

By assuming the role of the managing partner in the joint venture, the physician partners will gain professional autonomy of the work environment and the quality of care delivered to the patients. The group should have control over staffing decisions, equipment selection, purchasing decisions, and maintain direct influence over process and scheduling decisions. It is crucial for the joint venture to have a Director of Nursing in the administrative role, who has a knowledge of business as well as a strong clinical background to manage the joint venture. The Director should promote team work and have excellent communication and management skills, as well as an understanding of the difference in care delivery in an ambulatory surgery center setting versus an inpatient hospital setting.

Advantages of being the managing partner
Efficiency. The physician partner as the managing partner will be responsible for selecting anesthesia, administrative, nursing, and support staff that is qualified and capable of providing high quality care to the patients of the center. This staff is directly accountable to the physician partners for their performance. This staff works daily with the physician owners, which results in improved quality care for the patient. They all function as a team with one goal in mind: the delivery of high quality, safe, cost-effective care for the patient.

Increased productivity. Because of the efficiency of an ASC, the usual result is increased productivity for the physicians. The main reason for this is faster turn-over times. This allows the physician surgeons to complete their cases quickly, thus allowing them to complete larger case loads. Control of the surgical schedule also contributes to increased productivity. Outpatient procedures are elective procedures, rather than emergent, and therefore can be scheduled in advance for maximum efficiency and flexibility. The increase in surgical efficiency may also allow the physician to increase their revenue when more time is available to see more patients in the clinic setting. This may also expand the potential caseload for procedures to be performed in the ASC for both partner owners. As a result, both owners earn incremental income for each surgical procedure they perform by capturing the facility fee for each procedure.

Cost containment and standardization. By having control of equipment and supply selection decisions, the physicians can ensure they have modern technology available to serve their patient needs. The result of this yields patient access to improved services. Physicians also have the potential to standardize the supplies used for procedures, which will help reduce the procedure costs and improve revenues. By having the physician group determine what supplies are used, surgeon frustrations are eliminated, which normally emanate from hospital purchasing departments and budgeting politics, deciding what can and cannot be performed.

Satisfaction and high-quality care. The two most common reasons that patients state they prefer an ASC to a hospital are better service and more convenience. The managing partner can streamline the admission and discharge process, as well as make changes to protocols and practices as needed without having to go through committees and other administrative hurdles commonly seen in a hospital setting. New ideas for processes are therefore introduced and initiated more easily. The managing physicians work closely with staff that will provide direct input for change. By being accessible and working directly with the staff, a level of trust and camaraderie will develop. The end result becomes loyalty to the center, which in turn promotes efficiency, increased productivity, and high staff satisfaction, as well as superior patient care and patient satisfaction.

Staffing (nonunion and contract facility). The managing partner has the ability to maintain the joint venture as a nonunion or noncontract facility. This is especially important if the partner is a contract hospital, and the ASC has been established in a heavily unionized environment. If the managing partner has a union or contract base already established in their facility, this can filter into the new joint venture. Unionized staff within the center requires a whole new set of rules that must be complied with. Keep in mind that if the joint venture is built in an area where unions function, and the nursing population from which staff will be obtained is organized and functioning under a global contract, the owners must remain competitive when offering wages and benefit plans if the group wants to attract and retain skilled employees.

Disadvantages of being the managing partner

Two disadvantages to being the managing partner are:

- The physician partner must have established, within their own practice, efficient departments for collecting revenues, managing personnel, and have developed a human resource department.
- The physician partner will need to have a Director of Nursing who has a knowledge base of state and federal laws to maintain compliance with the rules and regulations for owning and operating an ASC.

Shared investment and risk

There are several advantages to partnering with a hospital or a corporate partner, from the physician partner's perspective: convenient location for the surgeons and patients, potential beneficial supply and services contracting, access to hospital's payer contracts, access to a certificate of need if required and, in many cases, a higher facility fee reimbursement. It is crucial that each partner has an equal investment and therefore ownership in the new joint venture. Even though the physician partner has equal investment risk, the physician must be the managing partner. Furthermore, the physician partner should negotiate a reasonable management fee for performing this service.

Supply and services contracting

Having a hospital or a "for profit" ASC corporation for a partner can be very beneficial when it is time to make capital purchases. Once the group has decided on the equipment and supplies necessary to set up the ASC, the group can access already established contracts for purchasing. The potential exists to save the joint venture significant amounts of money. The physician owner should be able to access the hospital's contract pricing for all of its purchases, including major equipment and instrumentation, as well as consumable supplies needed to complete the surgical caseload. This in turn will help reduce the cost of the surgical procedure, ultimately reducing over-all cost to the payers.

Payer contracts

The new joint venture, which includes a hospital partner, may be eligible for the same rate facility fees that the hospital already has negotiated with its payers. A major advantage to having a hospital partner will be having experienced personnel negotiating payer contracts. When the partnership negotiates with payers for inclusion of the new joint venture for facility fee reimbursements, experienced negotiators should assist in this process. This pre-existing relationship may expedite the ASC's ability to obtain contracts. If Medicare licensure and payer contracts have not been obtained before opening the ASC, there may be no patient volume to obtain cash flow. Most payers base their reimbursement on a percentage of Medicare. (Access the Federated Ambulatory Surgery Association Web site at www.fasa.org and click on CMS update or the CMS Web site at www.cms.hhs.gov.)

Access to legal counsel

After creating the joint venture, the physician owner may need access to legal counsel, whereas the hospital partner (or a "for-profit" corporate partner) may have their own established legal department. The hospital partner can then complete all the legal work, prepare all the documentation, and file all the paper work to establish the joint venture. By allowing the hospital partner to organize and prepare these documents, the physician partner should incur less cost. However, the physician group should have its own legal council look over all documentation to make sure that the physician partner is listed as the managing partner and that all expenses, voting rights, Board of Directors, governance, and shares are equally divided between partners. This may be the only opportunity to insure that all the terms and conditions of the contract are appropriate.

Training and education

It is well known that ASCs are efficient, productive environments to work in. This is because of the ability to have all staff members crossed-trained to be able to service the different subspecialties within the center. One of the disadvantages of an ASC may be its inability to have its own education and training department. This is an additional area where an established hospital or corporate partner may be advantageous. All major hospital systems have their own education center. The partnership can use this resource when mandatory training is necessary for basic life support, advanced cardiac life support, and radiation training, as well as other required state and federal mandatory training needs. The physician partner may use this knowledge base and adapt it to their own practice setting. Using this training center will save the joint venture money by not having to out-source it to a third party.

Potential cons of the ASC joint venture

The disadvantages of a joint venture, from a shared investment or risk point of view, include the following:

- The physician group must remember when entering into the joint venture that the physician partners must be the managing partner.
- The joint venture has the potential to be managed similarly to a hospital, if the physician partner is not the managing partner. Hospitals and corporate owners usually want majority ownership and control over the joint venture. If this happens, they will manage the venture like an inpatient hospital setting. This can lead to loss of efficiency, lower production, and loss of control. The original vision of the joint venture will change over time as the ownership and administration of the hospital changes and their vision for the center changes. This has the potential of the physician partner possibly losing control of the ASC.
- If the hospital is the managing partner in the joint venture, the center will be competing for capital dollars with the main hospital system. All revenue earned from the joint venture will be accessible to the entire hospital system. This will in turn reduce the physician group's profit margin, even though the physician partner has been efficient and maintained control of costs.
- If the partnership has been established with equal ownership, both partners will receive equal profit distribution. The number of procedures produced from the hospital partner must be monitored. Even though the hospital partner receives 50% of the profit from the joint venture, they may not be using the center to the same extent that the physician partners are. Furthermore, the hospital partner may not be contributing procedures which produce similar revenue profit margins. They may actually be sending to the facility their "loss leaders," or cases that produce little, if any, revenue. The physician managers will want to make sure that there is an increase in patients sent from the referral sources. It is difficult to enforce the usage of the center upon the hospital partner, and is almost impossible to force the hospital partner to take their "loss leaders" elsewhere, once they have established a schedule within the center. A fair management fee, established in the management agreement, may off-set some of the hospital partner's poor case mix. A fair management fee should include all of the medical group's costs of management, billing, and collections, and may include a stipulated share of revenues collected. As schedule of average nationwide management fees may be obtained from the Medical Group Management Association

and may be helpful in negotiating an advantageous management fee rate.

Summary

The key to any joint venture is in establishing who the managing partner will be. In an ASC joint venture, the physician partner is the most appropriate manager to run an efficient, productive, cost-effective, high-quality center. Having the physician group as the managing partner results in increased patient and staff satisfaction, and allows the group to hire experienced registered nurses, aides, and ancillary staff with appropriate social skills. There is no one better qualified to do this than the physician partner's management team, because they are in contact with the staff on a daily basis. Hospital administrators and managers are often out of touch with patient care simply because they do not perform any of it! Furthermore, they tend to be set in a particular management style and are unable to adapt to a progressively changing surgery center environment, with constantly changing payer expectations and technologic advances. The physician partner should always be attempting to contain cost, improve efficiency, and promote staff satisfaction, which will lead to increased productivity, as well as safe, efficient, high quality patient cares.

There are many advantages to a joint venture but there are also multiple risks. It is crucial to understand the advantages and disadvantages of this type of relationship before considering entering into it. For a list of organizations offering further research related to the advantages and disadvantages of joint venturing a surgery center, the following Web links may be of assistance:

http://www.outpatientsurgery.net/builders/2004/asc
http://www.fasa.org/
http://www.google/pros/cons/joint venture ambulatory surgery center

Further reading

FASA. Physician-led Ambulatory Surgical Centers Vital to Meeting the Surgical Needs of Tomorrow. January 2005.
Outpatient Surgery Magazine. The Wall Street View of Surgical Centers. Ryan S Daniels, CFA Chicago, January 2006.
Socioeconomic & Politics. Practice Management; The Pros and Cons of Developing an Ambulatory Surgery Center. November/December 2003.
Staunton EW, Vick JC. ASC business models: which one is right for you? Outpatient Surgery Magazine January 2004.

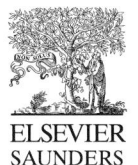

Developing an Orthopedic Ambulatory Surgery Center

Daniel A. Buehler, AIA[a], Trenton R. Mattison, MHA[b], Dana E. Mayberry, BS[a],*

[a]AmSurg, 20 Burton Hills Boulevard, Suite 500, Nashville, TN 37215, USA
[b]AmSurg, 3030 LBJ Freeway, Suite 700, Dallas, TX 75234, USA

Why consider owning a surgery center?

The following probably will not surprise a an orthopedic surgeon practicing in today's challenging health care environment:

- The Medical Group Management Association (MGMA) reports that although orthopedic practice revenues are generally rising, so are expenses. According to data from the MGMA's *Cost Survey for Orthopedic Practices: 2006 Report Based on 2005 Data*, almost 45 cents of each revenue dollar is consumed by practice overhead expenses [1].
- In a 2004 Orthopaedic Physician Census, the American Academy of Orthopaedic Surgeons/American Association of Orthopaedic Surgeons (AAOS) found that more 90% of the respondents in private practice agreed that practice expense increases and insurance reimbursement levels were among their most pressing concerns [2].
- Between 2004 and 2005, personal income decreased for one-third of the respondents to AAOS's 2006 Orthopaedic Physician Census [3].

In this environment of increased costs and constrained revenues/income, ancillary ventures such as orthopedic ambulatory surgery centers (OASCs) are crucial for orthopedic surgeons. An ownership interest in an OASC provides a new source of income, from facility fees, to supplement declining professional fees. According to the 2002 report of the MGMA annual cost survey, orthopedic practices with surgery centers offset the higher associated costs (for example, additional staffing needs in the center) with higher overall net profits than comparable practices without surgery centers [4]. Orthopedic practices with a surgery center also reported higher total medical revenue per physician than practices without a surgery center [4]. Owning an OASC provides additional income from the surgical cases the orthopedist already is performing and should be part of his or her future.

In addition to its financial benefits to orthopedic surgeons, OASCs can provide high quality, cost-effective, and efficient patient care. With the shift to consumer-driven health care, patients are playing an increasing role in making choices and directing their own health care dollars. An OASC can provide a practice with an attractive draw for these "empowered patients" by differentiating the practice in the marketplace. The patient-centered conveniences of an OASC will appeal to patients who will require outpatient surgical procedures.

Single-specialty advantages

When one considers the development of an ambulatory surgery center (ASC), the merits of a dedicated single-specialty orthopedic center versus a multispecialty center and the hospital outpatient department are clear. The advantages of a single-specialty center begin with the group of physician-owners. One may choose to develop a center solely with the surgeons in one's own

* Corresponding author. AmSurg, 20 Burton Hills Boulevard, Suite 500 Nashville, TN 37215.
 E-mail address: dmayberry@amsurg.com (D.E. Mayberry).

0030-5898/08/$ - see front matter © 2008 Elsevier Inc. All rights reserved.
doi:10.1016/j.ocl.2007.09.002

orthopedic.theclinics.com

practice or come together with like-minded physicians in the community. If one limits the scope of the center to orthopedics and the physician ownership group to orthopedic surgeons, one still can have enough projected volume to make the project feasible without diluting ownership across larger groups of specialists and specialties. With fewer owners in the OASC, each physician's share of the facility fee income will be greater.

A single-specialty OASC also will enhance productivity in numerous ways. Physicians using the surgery center will have more control over their own surgical schedules than in the hospital outpatient department, because surgeries and procedures in the OASC can be scheduled in advance and are not "bumped" for emergency cases. If the OASC is practice-based, one can reduce or eliminate travel time to multiple sites for outpatient surgery. A practice-based OASC provides familiarity and convenience for patients and can be less stressful for them than navigating a hospital's complicated parking situation and multiple entrances. The surgery center staff is especially selected and trained for the orthopedic specialty, resulting in maximum efficiency and productivity. With the center configured and equipped solely for orthopedics, there can be faster turnaround time between cases. The dedicated OASC also averts the "competition" with other specialties for operating rooms, staffing, and supplies that can arise in the hospital outpatient department or multispecialty surgery center.

For these reasons, a single-specialty OASC enables the orthopedist to perform more surgeries and procedures in less time. Beyond clinical training and expertise, time is the orthopedist's single greatest asset. Saving time and maximizing productivity with a single-specialty OASC results in additional professional time to provide quality care for current patients and to build a practice with new patients. It also can allow additional personal time for family, friends, and free-time pursuits.

In addition to allowing time savings, OASCs tend to be a lower-cost setting for surgeries, which is preferable to payors and patients. The co-insurance for Medicare patients, for example, is usually lower at an OASC than at a hospital outpatient department. Single-specialty surgery centers generally have significantly lower capital and operating costs than hospitals and multi-specialty-center alternatives, and these benefits can be passed on to payors and patients in lower-cost care. Payors in some states, such as South Carolina and New Jersey, reimburse for a site-of-service differential for cases performed in a surgery center rather than a hospital.

Despite the lower costs usually associated with OASCs, they also can be the location for the highest-quality patient care. At an OASC, orthopedic surgeons control the medical decisions. The center's layout and equipment are specific to orthopedic surgery. The physicians and the center's staff become expert in the repeat performance of the surgeries and procedures that are appropriately performed at the outpatient center. Numerous studies have suggested a link between higher volumes leading to higher proficiency and improved outcomes.

The combination of lower costs, superior quality, and convenience also will produce satisfied patients. A single-specialty OASC will thrive in the era of consumer-driven health care with its numerous patient-friendly amenities. Despite the laudable mission of hospitals, they often can be very daunting to patients. Patients will prefer the less institutional atmosphere of the OASC. The OASC will have a convenient location (particularly if it is practice-based) and simplified parking, especially compared with the usually Byzantine hospital complex. Patients will prefer the simplified admissions and discharge process. Patients also will benefit from the more predictable surgery schedule and will not have to fear getting "bumped" for urgent cases, as they might in the hospital. Because of potential overcrowding at the hospital, patients also might benefit from decreased waiting times. The surgery center staff tends to have higher job satisfaction, resulting in more pleasant interactions with the OASC patients.

Orthopedic ambulatory surgery centers versus specialty hospitals

Some orthopedic surgeons might consider development and ownership of an orthopedic specialty hospital instead of an OASC. Opponents of specialty hospitals are numerous, however, and therefore the political environment for developing an OASC is considerably less risky.

An orthopedic specialty hospital, by definition, allows surgeons to treat inpatients as well as outpatients. Proponents of specialty hospitals can make arguments about efficiency and quality similar to those of the developers of specialized surgery centers. They encounter outspoken opposition when the physician ownership component is added to the specialty hospital development, however.

Under federal Stark regulations regarding self-referral prohibitions, physicians are not allowed to invest in hospital departments and can invest only in the "whole hospital." Specialty hospital developers use this whole-hospital exception to allow physician ownership in these facilities.

Concerned that specialty hospitals might pose an economic threat to general hospitals, hospital lobbyists and some policymakers have diligently fought against them. In the Medicare Prescription Drug Improvement and Modernization Act of 2003, Congress enacted an 18-month moratorium on the development of new specialty hospitals and required both the US Government Accountability Office (GAO) and MedPAC (which advises Congress on Medicare and Medicaid issues) to conduct studies on the issue during that time. These studies suggested there might be unintended economic incentives in the Medicare payment system that encourage physician ownership in these facilities and that should be addressed with payment reforms.

The moratorium officially expired in June 2005, but the Centers for Medicare and Medicaid Services (CMS) essentially prolonged it by postponing the certification of new specialty hospitals while reviewing its procedures for enrollment. In light of the results of the GAO and MedPAC studies, the CMS delayed certifying new specialty hospitals to investigate the proportion of inpatient to outpatient cases at operational specialty hospitals. The CMS was concerned that some specialty hospitals with a high ratio of outpatient cases might be more similar to ASCs and be certified as specialty hospitals mostly to receive higher hospital outpatient department payment rates. In the Deficit Reduction Act of 2005, Congress advised CMS to consider collecting information on physician ownership of specialty hospitals. In 2007, the CMS proposed a new data collection effort (the "Disclosure of Financial Relationships Report") to aid in the analysis of hospital ownership structures and compliance with physician self-referral laws.

With such ongoing regulatory scrutiny, an orthopedic specialty hospital with physician ownership appears to have an uncertain future. By contrast, physician ownership in an OASC has better stood the test of time. Medicare began coverage for services provided in ASCs in 1982, and there are currently more than 4700 Medicare-certified ASCs in the country. Developing an orthopedic surgery center provides an orthopedist with the advantages of specialization and efficiency and seems to be far less politically risky.

Initial steps in developing an orthopedic surgery center

Feasibility analysis

The first step in developing an orthopedic surgery center is analyzing its feasibility. One must determine the number of physicians who will be using the facility and get verifiable historical procedure volume data from each (preferably from billing system reports). One must determine the percentage of procedures that are "movable" to the OASC. The CMS currently publishes a list of procedures that can be performed on Medicare patients in the ambulatory setting (available online at http://www.cms.hhs.gov/ASCPayment/), which can serve as a starting point in determining appropriate outpatient procedure volume.

One also must determine the procedure mix of the participating physicians, because it will influence the OASC design and profitability. The most commonly performed outpatient orthopedic procedures are knee arthroscopy, carpal tunnel release, and rotator cuff repair (although this mix might change with recent research indicating that exercise therapy produced outcomes comparable with surgery in patients who had rotator cuff impingement). One should not overlook the financial impact of implant costs. In general, reimbursements have not kept up with rising implant costs. In 2008, the CMS will begin implementation of a new phased-in ASC payment system tied to the hospital outpatient prospective payment system. The new system is expected to improve orthopedic payment rates and to better address implant costs.

The historical payor mix of the participating physicians also will affect the feasibility of the OASC project. How likely are payors to contract with the new OASC? Participating in payor networks is essential to the center's long-term survival, because obtaining reimbursement for out-of-network procedures is increasingly more onerous. Physicians who have heavier concentrations of patients enrolled in Medicare and health maintenance organizations should consider carefully their typically lower reimbursement rates. Physicians who have large volumes of worker's compensation cases also should be aware of any special issues or potential changes in payment systems. For example, changes in worker's compensation rules in California dramatically reduced reimbursements and raised the issue of physician self-referral.

One also must conduct a thorough market and competition analysis. Who are the other orthopedic surgeons in the area, and where do they perform their outpatient surgeries? Are there other OASCs or multispecialty surgery centers in the area, and where are they located?

The orthopedist probably will be moving cases from the hospital outpatient department to the new OASC. What are the current hospital politics in the area? How will the move affect the relationship with the hospital? At this point, it might be wise to remember that orthopedic surgeons represent an important revenue stream to the hospital, particularly for their inpatient cases. According to the hospital chief financial officers who responded to Merritt, Hawkins & Associates' 2007 Inpatient/Outpatient Revenue Survey, each full-time equivalent orthopedic surgeon was expected to produce an average of $2.3 million in net inpatient and outpatient revenue for the surveyed hospitals in 2007 [5]. Although a new OASC will begin to capture a small portion of this facility revenue with outpatient cases, the hospital will continue to receive the larger portion of the orthopedist's inpatient revenues. The hospital also might benefit from the efficiencies realized with a new OASC: with increased professional time to see new patients, it is possible that an orthopedist's inpatient work will increase.

In addition to calculating potential revenues, one also must estimate center development costs. A typical OASC with two operating rooms will require approximately 5000 square feet of usable area. Of course, local and state licensure standards will directly affect the size and, ultimately, the cost of the center, so care should be taken to engage an experienced design team to target the project's programmatic requirements and size specifically. A reasonable "median" cost for planning purposes would be $200 per square foot, which would include the buildout cost of the tenant improvements (not the shell of the building, site, or parking lots) and associated design fees. As with the square footage, this cost should be used only for planning purposes and should validated by local professionals with knowledge of the specific construction market. Costs will be higher in densely populated urban areas; in some suburban markets around the country, costs per square foot may be more competitive. The $200 is a target number that should be refined and reviewed as one progresses through the planning process and refines building program and plans. Equipment for a two-operating-room OASC will cost in the neighborhood of $1.5 million, including medical equipment, instruments, cleaning equipment, movable fixtures, and furniture. One also should factor in a working capital budget to cover center expenses for at least 6 months to a year while the new center is ramping up.

Legal and regulatory issues

There are innumerable legal and regulatory issues for a physician-owned surgery center, all of which require the assistance of an attorney with health care transaction experience to navigate. For example, the federal government and some states have rules governing physician self-referral. Federal Stark regulations do not define an ASC as one of the "designated health services" to which physicians are prohibited from referring their own patients if they have an ownership interest in the entity providing the service. Government enforcement of the Stark regulations, however, continues to clarify their meaning and intent, and it is absolutely necessary to understand and monitor those regulations. Additionally, the physicians and the surgery center entity must be in compliance with the federal (and some states') anti-kickback statute, prohibiting remuneration for referrals, as well as in compliance with Health Insurance Portability and Accountability Act (HIPAA) privacy rules.

There also are numerous legal and regulatory issues governing the development of the new OASC. Nearly half of all states still have certificate of need regulations that require approval from a designated state health-planning agency for new center construction (as well as for the expansion of existing centers). Each state has building licensure rules and requirements for the new OASC, and state licensure generally is required to participate in Medicare and Medicaid.

Partnership/ownership options

When deciding to develop a new OASC, one also must consider ownership options. Orthopedic surgeons have developed and managed surgery centers on their own, but doing so requires a significant investment of time, research, and capital from each of the physician-owners. Without the benefit of specific surgery center experience, physician groups run the risk of serious design problems, project delays, and cost overruns. When a physician group borrows money to develop the center itself, most banks will require each physician to provide joint and several guarantees on 100% of the borrowed amount. This requirement will significantly impact the physician's ability to borrow additional funds until this debt is retired.

Partnering with the local hospital is also an option. The hospital may have access to capital and may have payor relationships that can benefit the new OASC. Frustrations with the local hospital and its administration, however, often are the impetus for physicians to develop their own facilities. Although the hospital may be excellent at providing inpatient care, that ability does not necessarily translate into the expertise necessary to develop and manage an ASC. The OASC will not be the same as a hospital outpatient department and should not be managed in the same manner.

Physicians also can hire a consultant to assist in developing the new OASC. It is essential to determine the consultant's experience in specific surgery center development—it is not enough to have general health care experience. Most consulting companies are comprised of a small staff attempting to address the myriad issues involved in developing a center, as well as serving existing projects and recruiting new clients. Most consultants do not have access to significant capital. In general, consultants have a short-term perspective of a project (seeing it to completion), and their interests may not be in alignment with those of the physician-owners. Development consultants make their money whether the center that is developed performs at its potential or not.

Physicians also may choose to take on an equity partner in the new OASC. Corporate partners, such as AmSurg, with significant financial resources and extensive surgery center experience can provide capital and expertise in the development of an OASC. With "skin in the game" by investing in the surgery center development, the corporate partner's interests are in alignment with those of the physician-partners. It is in the best interests of both parties for the surgery center to be developed and to operate in the most efficient manner to maximize returns. In the ideal situation, the physician-owners and corporate partner have an equal voice in the governance of the surgery center and the decisions regarding its development and management. In a true collaboration, the corporate partner oversees the business aspects of the surgery center (including business office, marketing, financial reporting, accreditation, and administrative operations), while the physicians are freed to concentrate on providing superior patient care.

The center development process

Site location

Clearly the first and primary consideration for site location is proximity to the patient population. Sometimes one has an innate sense of where one's patients are coming from, which can be substantiated through a zip code analysis of the patient records. In many communities, however, population growth patterns should be considered so that the center can be well positioned for future population growth and change. A 5-year horizon is a good yardstick with which to judge potential locations as new communities are developed, roads and access constructed (or changed), and other shifts in growth occur.

In considering of the needs of the patient population (often older and/or infirm), some very basic and common sense issues should be evaluated. Is this a site where patients will recognize the address? Is this site easy to get to (interstate access, secondary roadway access)? Are there local landmarks that make the site easy to find? Can the site be accessed easily (right turn in, left "protected" turn lane)? Is the site easy to see from the roadway? What else is in the neighborhood (compatible use versus incompatible use or undesirable neighbors)? Is this site accessible by public transportation (particularly important in urban areas)? Will the necessary number of parking spaces fit on the site (usually in excess of what the local zoning regulations require)? In special consideration for orthopedic patients, is the space on the first floor and easily accessible by wheelchair?

Once a site is located, careful consideration should be given to the real estate entity that is created to own the land and the shell building (the landlord). If the landlord will be composed of the physician-partners in the surgery center, the composition of ownership is particularly important, especially if the real estate partnership does not mirror the surgery center partnership in its individual participants. The resultant disparity between "landlord" participants and "tenant" participants sometimes can lead to strains in relationships related to the real estate investment.

This distraction of energy and emotion is unnecessary and sometimes is dangerous to the newly formed surgery center entity. Clearly crafted "buy-in" and "buy-out" provisions should be created for the real estate component.

Design

The next step is design and construction. If a new building is to be constructed, it is very important to pay close attention to the design and cost of the shell building (as differentiated from the tenant's improvements), because these elements will drive the "base rent" requirement. As with any real estate transaction, control must be exercised to ensure a "market deal" to allow the economics of the overall surgery center to remain successful. If the shell building is constructed in a manner that drives the project costs higher than typical, the base rent to cover these costs will be higher. It is important that a market evaluation be done to ensure an "arm's length" transaction is being established with the landlord, or the surgery center will bear a rent structure higher than might be available by simply leasing space from a third-party landlord. Separating the landlord's and the tenant's responsibilities and scope of work/construction is important also. This separation of the shell building from the tenant improvements requires careful scrutiny and clear documentation from the very early stages of the project.

Selection of the design team for the surgery center is critical. Finding an architecture/engineering team with specific ASC experience is very important. Too little experience is one primary concern. "Other medical experience," although helpful, may be irrelevant. Having "designed my practice" is certainly irrelevant experience. Surgery center regulation and construction requirements are very specific to the development of a surgery center and are very specific to the orthopedic specialty. Underdesign or poor initial design will show up as regulatory comments/changes to the plans, change orders during construction, and/or failure of the facility during licensure and certification surveys before opening.

At the other end of the design spectrum, having a design team with only acute-care hospital experience is another concern. An excellent "hospital architect" will have superior knowledge of the acute-care regulatory environment and perhaps a working knowledge of surgery centers, but not enough. Overdesign of the surgery center environment will manifest as a facility that is too large, incorporating elements in the design that are excessive and not required for the surgery center, and ultimately will result in higher construction costs.

Having a lead architect with health care experience and specific surgery center experience will make the entire design and construction process move more quickly and will provide a more complete and accurate final product. Engaging an architect with clear knowledge of state regulations is an absolute necessity. It is also an advantage if the individual lead architect has some personal familiarity with the state agency regulators—and many do.

Compatible neighbors in the surgery center project is a plus, especially as related to co-location of the physician practice adjacent to the surgery center. Co-location of the practice facilitates patient convenience, physician convenience, and staff convenience and potentially lowers the overall per square foot cost of the project. Additionally, having compatible ancillary services as neighbors is an advantage: physical therapy/rehabilitation, imaging, and laboratory facilities adjacent to an orthopedic practice and surgery center provide the patient with a "one-stop shopping" experience. Combining all of these orthopedic services under one roof should enhance the ability to attract and serve the empowered patients in today's increasingly consumer-driven health care environment.

Construction

As with the design team, a general contractor who has specific experience in surgery center construction is strongly recommended. A surgery center is not a big doctor's office, nor is it a little hospital. Again, although "health care experience" is a plus, experience with surgery center construction is a significant advantage.

Engaging a contractor early in the design process is important for reasons of cost control and constructability review. Engaging a contractor who has surgery center experience also will reflect in accurate construction scheduling and schedule adherence. If one is adding to or renovating an existing surgery center, an experienced contractor also will assist with the critical issue of construction phasing, alternate work hours, and continuous infection control issues. Engaging the contractor as an early member of the design team also minimizes and sometimes can eliminate conflicts related to design flaws/missing design elements and associated change orders.

Equipment

An appropriate level of equipping is critical to the economic performance of the orthopedic surgery center. Overequipping (the center is not a hospital) can quickly destroy a budget and make the financial viability and performance of the surgery center a struggle for an extended period of time.

"Ramping up" equipment purchases over time, as the center's procedure volume ramps up, is recommended when it is possible to phase the purchase of equipment over time. Some equipment purchases may be made based on demonstrated need after the center is operational for some period of time, rather than making "safe" purchases based on the perceived need before the project opens. Clearly, a basic set of equipment is necessary for day-to-day operation upon opening, and an experienced architect, equipment planner, and/or clinical administrator can establish those criteria during the planning phase of the project. Establishing complete information about equipment needs early in the project process also will set a foundation for a successful economic model for the center, with required adherence to the equipment list.

Many staff members hired to work in a new center are new to the surgery center environment, with some coming from an acute-care hospital background. Operating in the surgery center environment is different and requires/allows a different use of equipment. When planning the equipment for a new surgery center, these staff members may need to compromise or adjust to using the equipment list that is generated for the center.

Policies and procedures

Documentation of clear, concise, and complete policies is mandatory. Clinical procedures must be documented, along with the steps taken to maintain the quality of the environment (eg, filter changes, exercising generator). Policies also will include agreements with outside services for clinical operations (eg, hospital transfer agreement), as well as physical plant operations (eg, cleaning and biohazard handling).

Mapping individual policies to each element of the state licensure law and to the Medicare regulations is a necessity. These regulations are the yardstick with which the licensure and certification agencies will measure the completeness of the center's policies.

Several accrediting bodies also promulgate standards for achieving approval under their jurisdiction. Their respective accreditation requirements can be an excellent tool in establishing and measuring the appropriateness and completeness of the center's policy and procedure manual.

Licensure and certification

To receive Medicare payment for services provided in the surgery center, Medicare requires that "the OASC must comply with State Licensure requirements" as a condition of coverage (Section 416.40). As such, many of the physical facility requirements for the surgery center are found in the state's licensure laws. With a few exceptions, the Medicare certification requirements are silent on most facility issues, incorporating the state licensure laws by reference. One should not spend a lot of time poring through the Medicare requirements to find what size the operating room must be. In addition, one should be skeptical if one hears, "… because it's required by Medicare…" if the comments are related to size, number, and/or types of spaces and their attributes.

Many states have adopted the *AIA Guidelines for Construction and Equipment of Health Care Facilities* (or some form thereof) as an element of their licensure requirements. Some states have guideline documents that are parallel to the AIA guidelines, and some states have written the language of the guidelines into their state's building code. In all cases, the licensure standards are where all of the physical requirements of the surgery center can be found: the number of spaces, their size, their orientation to one another, and the services available to them (eg, medical gases, emergency power, HVAC requirements).

The architect's first step in the design process should be to contact the state and determine what rules and regulations are in effect and what version (the year or edition) of the AIA guidelines have been adopted. The architect also should determine what process the licensure agency will follow during the plan review stage and how long the process will take. Some states have an expedited review process, but others may take as many as 6 months or more to review and approve plans for construction. One should learn of this schedule early in the process, because it affects everything else that happens for the duration of the construction project. In addition, the design/build team should clearly determine the survey and review process to which the project will be subject during construction, because it will vary by state.

Finally, the team should be familiar with the time frames, scheduling requirements, and filing and administrative process at the close of the project's construction to determine the timeline for licensure surveys and subsequent Medicare certification surveys. Once state licensure is obtained, Medicare may directly survey the facility, typically using the same team of surveyors from the state, and grant certification if the center passes. Alternatively, Medicare may award the new center certification without a Medicare survey by "deemed status," if the facility is surveyed and passes accreditation by one of the national, Medicare-approved accrediting bodies that have been granted "deeming" powers.

Managing the operational center

Once the challenges of designing, building, and equipping a surgery center within state regulations and federal requirements have been met, managing the business begins. Preparing for managing the facility should not be taken any more lightly than the development phase. The regulatory environment is very complex, with state licensure and Medicare certification requirements and increasing administrative burdens ranging from Stark laws to HIPAA requirements. A highly specialized management team is needed to navigate this regulatory environment, and the time commitment can be very burdensome for a physician practice to manage alone. The initial management challenges include staffing and managed care contracting.

Staffing

A primary objective to achieving the center's mission of low-cost, high-quality care is adequate and controlled staffing and scheduling. Staffing a surgical team dedicated to one specialty creates maximum staff efficiency, expertise, and productivity. With a more predictable and preferred work schedule than at the hospital, the center staff has a higher degree of control and satisfaction in the delivery of care. Working together in the highly specialized OASC results in a high degree of familiarity and trust between the staff and physicians.

Nurses and ancillary staff are attracted to the OASC because of their desire to work in an environment where they can become experts in the delivery of highly specialized care and not take call. The OASC schedule is more predictable and controlled than the hospital setting. Therefore, proper staffing levels are more easily anticipated and maintained, with the need for less part-time staff than in the hospital. For these reasons turnover is historically much lower at ambulatory facilities than at more traditional inpatient facilities. A productive, stable, and happy staff translates to higher patient satisfaction with the center.

The most crucial hire for the new center is the director of nursing. The director of nursing will be the eyes and ears of the facility and ensure the mission of the facility is never compromised. The mission probably will encompass the objectives of serving the needs of the community in a low-cost, high-quality, comfortable, and convenient setting. The facility will be dedicated to patient-centered health care, without sacrificing a commitment to excellence in medical technology and treatment.

The center's management team must take steps to create and capitalize on the inherent staff efficiencies and productivity in the single-specialty surgery center setting. The center must offer continuing education and professional development activities, both to comply with licensure regulations and to keep its staff current on new technologies and best practices. Management must facilitate the relationship between staff and the physician-owners by encouraging the open communication and celebration of the center's successes. Creative incentive plans can motivate compliance to the highest standards.

An annual employee satisfaction survey can give center staff a mode of confidential communication with center management and the physician-owners. The survey results can be used for center improvements and to make everyone's jobs easier or more efficient. Surveying what motivates the staff is essential to developing a high-performance staff team.

Contracting

Obtaining and maintaining payor contracts (thereby attracting patients) for the new center can be a full-time job. The most important element in contracting is negotiating a fair reimbursement for the surgical procedures performed at the center, which requires a thorough understanding of the center's actual case costs. To enhance the center's ability to negotiate reimbursements, it is important to establish and maintain relationships with the individuals representing the payor in rate negotiations. Ongoing relationships with contracting, case management, and provider relations personnel at the various payors is vital for growing the surgery center business.

To negotiate contracts successfully, it is important to know the audience—to get to know them personally. Payors are more likely to work with someone they like and trust. Secondly, one should be their resource. Educating them on the benefits of contracting with and using the OASC and on the cost effectiveness of the OASC and its costs per procedure can facilitate rate negotiations. Offering center tours also can be beneficial in negotiating competitive rates. It is very powerful to have the payor representative tour the center because he or she will witness at first hand the comfort and convenience that the patients experience.

Future prospects

Once the properly developed and professionally managed surgery center is open for business, its future prospects look good. Continuing improvements in anesthesia and technology will continue to support the migration of surgical procedures to outpatient venues. Medical literature also reveals continuing improvements in minimally invasive surgical techniques and pain control, with the possibility of outpatient knee and maybe even hip replacements in certain patient populations.

With implementation of the new ASC payment system in 2008, the CMS will eliminate the list of procedures that can be performed on Medicare patients in a surgery center. Historically, the CMS was not able to provide timely and appropriate updates to this list of covered procedures, thereby limiting services to Medicare patients. In its place, there will be a much shorter list of procedures that the CMS deems unsuitable for the surgery center. This change will open up the range of clinically safe and appropriate surgeries available to Medicare patients in an OASC.

Demographics also point to a likely increase in demand for orthopedics. The "baby boom" generation, which has transformed each age group progressively, is not expected to age quietly. Rather, most Boomers will seek to maintain their active lifestyles with attendant orthopedic trauma and injuries. Patients already are requiring joint replacement at earlier ages, and the likelihood of repeat procedures increases as the replaced joints themselves need replacing.

Baby Boomers probably will continue to demand amenities and conveniences like no generation before them, a demand that is contributing to the empowered consumer transformation in health care. An OASC, with its emphasis on patient convenience and satisfaction as well as quality care, should become a preferred location for those Boomers requiring orthopedic surgery services.

Summary

Although there are risks, the potential benefits should encourage orthopedists to consider developing an OASC. The demands of developing the OASC, as well as having it operate efficiently, are complex and time-consuming. There are, however, experts that can assist in developing and managing a highly efficient center, freeing the orthopedist to concentrate on performing surgery in an environment that is clinically, financially, and personally rewarding. Patients should appreciate the numerous care enhancements they experience at a surgery center. The orthopedist can enjoy the benefits of increased income with the revenues from surgery center ownership and the time savings and productivity enhancements provided by the surgery center. Overall, an OASC is an excellent investment in the future.

References

[1] Fisher SE. Orthopaedic revenues and expenses keep increasing. American Association of Orthopaedic Surgeons Bulletin, July 2007. Available at: http://www.aaos.org/news/bulletin/jul07/managing10.asp. Accessed October 9, 2007.

[2] Porucznik MA. 2004 Orthopaedic Physician Census results released. American Association of Orthopaedic Surgeons Bulletin, February 2005. Available at: http://www2.aaos.org/aaos/archives/bulletin/feb05/acdnws3.asp. Accessed October 9, 2007.

[3] Watkins-Castillo S, Porucznik MA. Measuring up: The 2006 Orthopaedic Physician Census. American Association of Orthopaedic Surgeons Bulletin, August 2006. Available at: http://www2.aaos.org/aaos/archives/bulletin/toc.cfm?IssueMonthName=August&IssueYear=2006. Accessed October 9, 2007.

[4] Redling R. Crunching numbers: Ancillary services on the rise. Medical Group Management Association e-Connexion, Issue 23, January 2003.

[5] Merritt, Hawkins & Associates. 2007 Physician Inpatient/Outpatient Revenue Survey. Available at: http://www.merritthawkins.com/pdf/2007_Physician_Inpatient_Outpatient_Revenue_Survey.pdf. Accessed October 9, 2007.

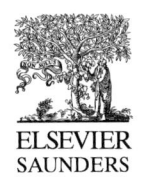

Financing and Cash Flow Management for the Medical Group Practice

Andrew J. Bert, BS, CPA, MST*

2519 Humboldt Avenue South, Unit 107, Minneapolis, MN 55405, USA

The expansion of a medical group practice and the addition of ancillary services require a substantial cash outlay. Obtaining proper financing to complete a successful expansion is a process that takes time, and there are critical steps that need to be followed. The group's business objectives must be presented properly by developing a business plan detailing the practice and goals associated with the desired expansion. A pro forma analysis must be developed that is conservative but reasonably accurate in projecting revenues, expenses, and cash flow related to the practice and planned expansion. Finally, developing a relationship with a reputable bank is necessary to facilitate construction and eventually completion of the desired expansion.

Business plan

Every company should have a business plan. The plan, in fact, should be a "work in progress," updated continuously and maintained as the practice expands. The purpose of the business plan is to function as a description of the group's business to outside sources; it will help the group's partners gain insight into the general structure of the business functions of the practice. This business plan needs to be developed before outside financing is obtained and can serve as a tool that will help determine the best available financial plan for the medical practice.

The business plan should contain the following items:

- Executive summary
- Medical practice description
- Medical business management organization
- Available Patient Products and services
- Physician and patient marketing plan
- Business operational plan
- Capitalization and structure
- Financial needs
- Financial plan
- Risk factors

This article discusses some of the key elements from this list that are essential in creating an overall effective business plan for the group medical practice.

Executive summary

The executive summary is one of the most critical aspects of the business plan. The summary should be concise in providing an overview of the plan as well as the practice goals. This summary initiates the business plan and should include the reasoning why practice growth and expansion is important.

After the business plan has been assimilated, it will be easier to summarize. Therefore, it usually is easier to write the summary after the business plan is completed. It is important to keep the executive summary brief and concise!

Practice description

The practice description should include information about the basics of the medical practice as well as the reasons why expansion of the medical practice will be successful and will help the practice grow fiscally. When describing the basics of the medical practice, be sure to explain the

---

* 3601 W 76th St., Edina, MN 55435.
E-mail address: andrew.bert@lacrosseglobal.com

demographics of the current practice patient base as well as plans for capturing future market share. Explain how the expansion will benefit these patients. This analysis should include a description of how the different elements of the practice, such as ancillary services and/or multiple offices, may provide better patient service and convenience. Because this practice evaluation must be presented to a financial institution to obtain a loan at a favorable rate, a positive evaluation of the future of the medical practice expansion is important. Often the pro-forma analysis based on a market analysis of the area can be developed to aid in the presentation to the lending institution.

Financing needs

The subsequent sections discuss some standard methods of obtaining financing for a medical practice that plans on adding ancillary services. As described in a later section, business as well as personal accounts should be established at the chosen lending institution, because doing so will help build a strong personal and business relationship and, as a result, obtain favorable lending rates.

Financial plan

This financial plan section of the business plan should include the medical group physicians' financial statements that the lending institution will require when a financing proposal is presented. Prior financial statements and tax returns usually are required for the last 3 business years for each physician personally, as well as their prior business financial statements and tax returns.

The most important part of this section is the pro-forma analysis, the analysis of prospective financial performance. This analysis is a necessary part of the financial evaluation that will need to be completed before even considering the business expansion.

Pro-forma analysis

Pro-forma analyses are critical when evaluating a prospective business venture and will help outline optimal operational and financing strategies for the medical practice expansion. Included in pro-forma analyses are revenue and expense projections as well as cash flow estimates. The cash flow approximations are essential in determining the overall financing structure. These projections should be conservative enough to include some practice development time to allow for the delay in revenue collection from the new practice expansion.

Revenue, expense, and cash flow should be projected out monthly for the first 12 to 18 months and then in yearly increments for 5 years. Technically, either the cash method or the accrual method of accounting may be used in presenting the pro-forma statements, but most financial institutions prefer the accrual method because more information can be relayed regarding the accounts receivable as well as accounts payable.

The key to developing an accurate pro-forma analysis is to generate a list of assumptions that will be used in developing the revenue model. Some assumptions that help develop revenue expectations are the timing of reimbursements, the demographics of the expected patient base, expected referral sources, the payer mix, and production estimates. Attention should be paid to both the payer mix and patient demographics. For example, if many of the expected patients are elderly, Medicare may be a significant payer, and the reimbursement rates may be significantly lower than with other payers. Expense estimates must be evaluated by paying attention to the staffing needs of the expansion. Although economies of scale may be realized as the practice expands, sufficient staffing needs and corresponding benefit expenses must be accounted for in cash flow estimates. Once the practice growth model is developed, the group must account for the correct payer contracts needed to realize expected revenues.

Most medical practices use the cash method of accounting in which revenues are not recognized until they are received. It may take 45 to 90 days to collect from payers. The banks may desire to view the pro-forma analysis based on the accrual method. This can be done by assuming a certain collection period, and then recognizing the revenue when it is collected. This article does not discuss the details of how to utilize the accrual method of accounting, but it may be desirable to take this delayed collection period into consideration in estimating cash flow projections when developing the pro-forma analysis. A medical practice's revenue is projected, starting with gross revenue and then subtracting the negotiated contractual discounts as well as subtracting an estimate of the uncollectible revenues. Contractual discounts usually run from 45% to 60%, so before any revenue projections are generated, it is imperative that the practice have a fair assumption of the contractual discounts.

Consultant advice will be needed to develop a realistic pro-forma analysis. Other medical groups who already have executed a similar expansion strategy can be a source of information. Business advisors with knowledge and experience in developing pro-forma analyses for medical practices involved in the development of ancillary services can be consulted. Equipment suppliers with whom the group has existing relationships also may help in estimating specific revenue, expense, and cash flow projections related to the acquisition and implementation of desired medical equipment. It is helpful to obtain opinions from a multitude of sources.

Capital

Determining how to fund the medical practice expansion will become easier once a detailed pro-forma analysis is developed that outlines what financing will be necessary. This financing can originate from several sources. Initially, a good banking relationship should be established with a line of credit at the optimal rate. A capital call structure may be established with the medical group partners if financing options are exhausted or if the partners are "risk averse" and do not want to be individually liable for large loan amounts. Often, the partners may wish to diversify and use multiple financing methods to minimize their risk exposure. Finally, if additional practice assets need to be acquired, another financing method is to enter into leasing contracts with the company that is providing the asset.

Bank relationship

As noted previously, a good banking relationship is important. The choice of bank is a critical decision that should be considered carefully. The local reputation of the bank as well as its financial performance and "net worth" should be evaluated. While the bank is evaluating the group's requests, the group should be evaluating the bank's financial statements. If the group practice "performs" for the bank with multiple loans from the bank to the group and its partners, the practice may need its help in the future for practice expansion. Often a bank that has experience in health care financing is more understanding of the process and will be easier to work with.

It may be better to utilize a bank that is somewhat smaller, in terms of net worth, because it may be more eager to develop a long-term relationship with a medical group. It is common for larger banking systems to be more hesitant to give preferred lending rates to a new medical group. The physicians within the group often would prefer to borrow from the bank to finance capital purchases rather than use cash that normally is distributed from their accounts receivable as salary.

It is important that the group ask for lines of credit for all the physicians individually. Doing so will help establish a firm relationship with the bank and usually results in preferred lending rates.

Banks will analyze the group's pro-forma analysis and will use this information to determine the earning potential of the practice. They also will focus on assets that they can secure or use as collateral should the practice be unable to service the debt. Personal guarantees may be another part of the equation that could be considered, depending on the amount of financing being requested and the collateral being used. Start-up ventures always are deemed to be risky ventures for a bank to finance, so a well-established practice will be viewed as a safer investment for the bank.

Capital call

Whether the doctors in the practice plan to invest capital in the expansion or already have capital invested in the practice is another aspect the banks will consider. This investment is termed a "capital call." A capital call means that each partner in the practice contributes an equal amount of capital to the practice to help finance the expansion. This scenario obviously is more viable if there is a greater number of doctors in the practice. Because some financing plans may require that each doctor have a significant investment as a partner in the practice, the doctors who have the highest net worth often are at the greatest risk. For this reason each doctor should have an individual entity set up to protect him or her individually from liability. This method of personal protection is termed "joint and several liability," which means that multiple individuals are liable for an obligation, such as a bank loan, for the practice.

Requiring that the doctors in the practice have an amount guaranteed or a certain amount invested in the practice provides an incentive to keep them all focused on the goal of developing the business. If an outside investor becomes involved in the medical practice, however, undue influence on the business model may develop, and financial problems can arise. The doctors involved should have a significant control of the medical and business aspects of the group practice. As more physicians become financially involved, risk of default is minimized. Often, involving different types of specialists (depending on the ancillary facility) can be helpful so that, if one specialty is not using the new facilities, others can help alleviate an unexpected downturn in revenue.

Equipment leasing and purchasing

The useful life of an asset should be analyzed when deciding to lease or purchase the asset. Equipment that is expected to last 10 to 15 years should be purchased if it fits within the group's financing plan.

Leasing can provide additional financing and should be considered when cash flow is tighter. Leasing is a viable option for a group that is just starting out and does not have the cash to purchase expensive equipment. The most common types of leases are operating leases and financing or capital leases. With an operating lease, the lease payments are treated as operating expenses. This lease provides a low cost of use, and the lease will not be accounted for on the balance sheet, meaning no asset or liability is recorded. The monthly payment is deducted, and at the end of the term of the lease the equipment will be returned to the lessor. The medical group then is free to lease or purchase new equipment. A capital lease allows the group to record the liability on the balance sheet and also allows the depreciation of the equipment to be deducted from the corporate profits. As with any other lease, there also is an option to purchase the equipment at a discount at the termination of the lease. Because a capital lease in essence allows the group to treat the equipment as though it were owned, the group is responsible for maintenance costs, taxes, and insurance.

If a group believes that it will need to upgrade equipment before the lease is over, it can terminate a lease early, but it still will be responsible for the remaining lease payments. For this reason it is essential to determine the useful life of the equipment. If it is expected that an upgrade may occur after only a few years of service, this likelihood should be considered when determining lease types and lease terms.

Leasing medical equipment has become a more popular trend recently, as illustrated by a study available at http://www.chooseleasing.org/market/MedSur.htm. This study explains that new technologies highly affect the need for new equipment and that customers value these new technologies. Also, the average lifespan for high-cost medical equipment is only approximately 5 years.

Although interest rates are important, the group should match its financing, which includes leasing of equipment, with the cash flow anticipated once the ancillary services are functioning. The ramp-up period may be unpredictable and can take up to 6 months; this period should be considered in estimating cash flow needs, because bank payments may occur within these first 6 months. The group's financing plan should allow for additional operating loans to avoid cash-flow problems within these first 6 months. The lending institution must understand that during the development period for the medical practice, when new ancillary services or a new practice location begins to function, it may take 90 to 180 days for reimbursements to occur.

Definitions

Capital or financing lease

A capital or financing lease is a lease that meets any of the following criteria:

- The lease term is greater than 75% of the property's estimated economic life.
- The lease contains an option to purchase the property for less than fair market value at the end of the lease term.
- The ownership of the property is transferred to the lessee at the end of the lease term.
- The present value of the lease payments exceeds 90% of the fair market value of the property.

Operating lease

An operating lease is any lease that is not a capital lease. An operating lease cannot have any of the criteria listed as necessary for a capital lease. Additional services such as maintenance and insurance can be provided by the lessor. Furthermore, the lease payments are tax deductible.

Recourse and non-recourse loans

Two types of financing loans are recourse and non-recourse loans. In recourse financing, if a practice defaults on the loan, the doctors are liable for payment to the lender. With non-recourse financing the borrower (the practice) is not liable if the practice defaults on a loan. The lender then can recover the amount owed by foreclosing on the property by which the loan is secured. Tax laws limit the amount of losses that can be claimed on a business investment to an amount at-risk on non-recourse debt.

In summary, important strengths to present when attempting to acquire financing are exhibiting superior management of the expansion facilities, a realistic pro-forma analysis with an appropriate market analysis for the practice's services, and a thorough explanation of why the practice needs enough liquidity until the ambulatory surgical center is able to establish a positive cash flow because of delayed reimbursement by Medicare and private insurers. Preparation of these elements is critical to obtaining a favorable result from a lending institution. Remember that the bank also has a tremendous amount to gain from developing a strong relationship with a successful medical group practice.

Acknowledgments

The author acknowledges the expertise of Farley Kaufmann, CPA, and Stacie Usem, CPA, and thank them for their suggestions in the development of the content of this article.

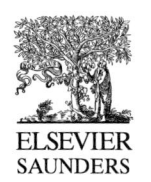

Gain-Sharing with the Hospital: What is Possible in the Current Legal Environment

Paul M. Torgerson, JD

Dorsey & Whitney LLP, Suite 1500, 50 South Sixth Street, Minneapolis, MN 55402, USA

Much of the health care delivery model in this country relies on the goodwill and cooperation of institutional providers, such as hospitals, and independent professional clinical providers who make up the medical staff. Often, institutional providers offer both inpatient and outpatient services while relying on a combination of employed professionals and independent medical staff members to deliver the professional physician component of the service. For simplicity, this article refers to "hospitals" rather than "institutional providers." Because the interaction between hospitals and physicians is often extensive, those interested in clinic management also must be knowledgeable about the hospital setting and the opportunities in these situations for improved clinic and physician performance.

Within hospital settings, patients expect that institutional processes and the clinical processes brought to the facility by the independent professionals will work together to produce quality outcomes. Hospitals, however, often are not in a position to mandate physician behavior, and independent physicians develop their own processes and expectations. Consequently, to the outside observer, the processes within a single service line, such as outpatient surgery, or in ancillary services such as imaging do not seem to be well aligned. In many cases, the hospital and physicians are not even pursuing the same goals for the service. This phenomenon often is described as "fragmented care," because there is not a single point of accountability for clinical and operational process outcomes.

For example, in pursuit of efficiency and cost-effectiveness, a hospital may be highly motivated to ensure that surgical cases start on time, that operating room turnaround time is as short as possible, and that staff time is not wasted. The independent physician may have a general desire to work toward those goals, but nothing in the environment incences a physician to pursue those goals actively, as opposed to the physician's goal of making his or her own time most productive, moving back and forth between the physician's own clinic and the hospital. The goals of the hospital and physician frequently are malaligned if not in conflict.

Similarly, a hospital's desire to provide efficient imaging services to both inpatients and outpatients frequently conflicts with the physician's desire to refer a patient to a service with the most convenience and speedy reporting of results. When a physician's patient referred to a hospital imaging service is bumped in favor of the more urgent need of an inpatient, the physician can feel that the patient has been ill served. It is not surprising that physicians will explore how they may be able to provide better the service themselves (possible injuring the hospital's profitability in the process) to increase patient convenience and expedite patient care.

Several other environmental factors add to the tension between hospitals and physicians. Through skill development, technology, and discovery, many care modalities have migrated in recent times from inpatient to outpatient settings, and the pace of migration continues to increase. Also, under heavy pressure from governmental and other payers to constrain payment for professional and hospital services, independent professionals constantly look for new ways to make

E-mail address: torgerson.paul@dorsey.com

up for reduced payments for their services. In many cases, physicians discover that in their clinic or other physician-owned settings they can provide services that only hospitals previously provided. These dynamics have resulted in a proliferation of physician-owned diagnostic facilities, surgery centers, and, more recently, specialty hospitals. Facing similar pressures, hospitals work hard to retain their ability to provide the outpatient services but frequently must rely on the very professionals who are driven to offer the service directly themselves. The tension of competing interests frequently weakens trust between hospital and physician.

Patients, meanwhile, often experience this environment as "fragmented care," which can be prone to error and patient dissatisfaction. Payers and the public observe duplication of cost, clumsy inefficiency in the medical records arena, and existing tension between the components of this fragmented system.

Realizing the competition for patients, hospitals have only a few realistic strategic approaches. They can fight physicians for dominance in a service line, duplicate resources and compete for staff, or hire physicians. They may yield ownership of ancillaries while trying to maintain positive relationships in the other professional service interactions within the hospital, or they can engage physicians actively in a joint exploration of process improvements, searching for ways to avoid duplication and waste of resources. Many institutions have attempted the first two approaches with varying degrees of success. This article focuses on the third category and, within that category, on the idea of gain-sharing, defined as engagement between the hospital and physicians to create effective joint processes, common outcome measures, joint accountability, and a sharing of results.

For a variety of reasons, some of which are described later in this article, the term "gain-sharing" has acquired a pejorative, almost suspicious connotation among the federal and state regulators who oversee health care delivery. Understood in light of the environment described previously, it should not be so. Gain-sharing is merely one logical approach to addressing fragmented care, cost containment, and improved clinical outcomes.

Any serious student of process improvement will realize the potential in bringing institutional and independent physician processes together into a fully aligned service offering. A number of elements are essential to achieving this potential, including common understanding of the environment and commitment to common goals, working together as a single team, jointly identifying opportunities and then tackling them together to increase effectiveness, and sharing in the results of the common work. If successful, such efforts reduce duplication of resources, heighten patient satisfaction, reduce costs, and enable clinical improvement while creating a more engaged and less frustrated workforce.

Gain-sharing is nothing more than a tool to bring about these results, a tool that gives physicians reasons to cooperate with hospitals—the potential for clinical improvement, seamless patient experiences, financial advantages, sharing of capital costs for ancillary services, and hope for a more satisfactory working environment through reduction in fragmentation. Additional motivation can be found in the demands from payers to report the clinical outcomes from the joint efforts of independent physicians and hospitals and in the widespread acknowledgment that fragmented care contributes to medical errors. Gain-sharing may be an important tool in improving the nation's health care delivery system.

All "phynancial" relationships are suspicious

Various attributes of the current health care system create the fear of abuse in gain-sharing programs. First, cost-reduction programs in which physicians share the results could create an inappropriate incentive for those physicians to reduce necessary medical care. Second, sharing improved financial results with physicians could create an incentive for physicians to overuse financially attractive services. Third, close financial relationships between a hospital and physician might result in decision-making based on the relationship rather than the best interests of the patient (eg, a physician might refer a patient to an inferior program because the physician has a close financial relationship with that program). Fourth, some observers regard a variety of close relationships merely as devices to redirect funds from institutions to physicians to ensure physician loyalty. That fear is even more ominous if one of the partners is tax-exempt and is seen as creating a device to share exempt earnings with a private party. It sometimes is suggested that physicians should undertake the improvement activities without any financial incentive to do so. That view, however, largely ignores the significant negative financial impacts imposed on physicians in recent decades of change.

Suspicions of financial relationships, together with other factors, have led to strict regulation of relationships between physicians and other health care providers. No one actively working in health care today is unaware of the Stark law, the Medicare anti-kickback law, the civil monetary penalties law, restrictions on tax-exempt organizations, and all the related complex regulations.

The current state of affairs

The term "gain-sharing" often is used to refer to any arrangement in which physicians and a hospital or other provider work together on a service line or cost-reduction project, including equity joint ventures, comanagement contracts, specific process improvement projects, and even some employment arrangements. This article focuses on contracts under which a hospital or institutional provider retains an independent clinic or physicians to tackle specific issues of service line performance.

The gain-sharing transaction

A gain-sharing program most often emanates from a review of a costly clinical program and realization that independent physicians control many hospital costs but have no accountability if those costs increase dramatically. Examples include opening sterilized packs during surgery, the contents of sterilized packs, determining what variety of devices must be maintained in inventory, and lack of coordination between anesthesia and surgeons in connection with start times and turn-around times in the operating room. Wide variation in physician practice can add dramatically to hospital costs. Both hospitals and physicians realize that cooperation is necessary to create common expectations and to motivate changes in physician behavior that could improve the patient experience and the performance of the service. Typically a hospital will identify the physicians who are in a position to seek improvement opportunities, whose cooperation is essential in delivering change, and whose leadership skills can effectively motivate others to execute the plans.

A hospital and physician group may enter into an agreement for the physician's time and effort in identifying improvement opportunities, benchmarking "best in class" clinical outcomes and service levels, developing appropriate clinical protocols, serving as a project team member, serving as liaison with other medical staff, driving changes in physician behavior among the professionals engaged in the service, and monitoring the results of actions taken. In some cases, the physician might have a direct role in the management of the service within the hospital. In a gain-sharing program, the compensation mechanism would include payment for the new management and administrative duties performed by physicians and also sharing of the benefits from a successful intervention. In short, the gain-sharing transaction attempts to align the clinical and financial interests of the parties.

Navigating the regulatory waters

As noted earlier, the financial and other relationships created in a gain-sharing program have the potential to create incentives that abuse patients by placing physician and hospital financial interests above patients' interests or that abuse government programs by using more services than necessary for physician and hospital financial gain. Specific statutes and related regulations prohibit certain behavior in these contexts:

Medicare anti-kickback laws [1]
Stark referral prohibitions [2]
Civil Monetary Penalty Law [3]
When a tax-exempt hospital is involved, tax-exemption requirements precluding inurement or private benefit are also implicated [4].

The views of responsible regulators in these areas have changed over time, and those views are not always in sync with one another. For example, the Internal Revenue Service initially had a favorable view of gain-sharing, then reversed itself; and then simply ceased issuing guidance on the subject. The Office of Inspector General (OIG) of the US Department of Health and Human Services initially rejected the idea but later approved a number of fairly restrictive arrangements in advisory opinions in the context of the Medicare anti-kickback and civil monetary penalties statutes [5,6]. The Centers for Medicare and Medicaid Services (CMS) has not directly tackled the issue under the Stark law, for which it has responsibility. In the current regulatory landscape, hospitals, and physicians perceive a chilling effect from the regulations, and gain-sharing transactions are pursued cautiously. It is important to monitor the regulatory landscape constantly, and it would be dangerous to develop a gain-sharing transaction without involving an attorney knowledgeable in these health care regulatory areas. Some transactions also may warrant seeking an advisory opinion from the regulators. Consequently, gain-sharing transactions can be expensive to develop.

Current framework for an approved gain-sharing program

Development of a gain-sharing program today requires an understanding of the feared abuses addressed through statutes and regulation and specific transaction features that prevent abuse from occurring. As of the date of publication, a program approved by regulators would include a combination of some or all of the following:

1. Limited duration of the agreement (an arrangement of 1 year has been approved by the OIG)
2. A detailed work-plan and job description sufficient to enable a determination that compensation paid under the program is fair market value
3. Independent medical confirmation that the program elements and protocols will not result in withholding of care
4. Effective documentation of savings achieved, using current costs as baseline
5. An effective means of de-linking the award from the volume or value of referrals made by any particular physician
6. A cap on the amount of the gain-sharing award (eg, 50% of documented savings)

Continuing evolution

Unlike the current public debate surrounding the origin of the universe, few in the health care field can find evidence of intelligent design in the make-up and nature of the health care system in the United States. Nevertheless, there is evidence of some ongoing effort to improve the environment for patients, physicians, and hospitals. In recent testimony to the Subcommittee on Health of the House Committee on Ways and Means, the Chief Counsel to the Inspector General of the US Department of Health and Human Services acknowledged the potential benefits of gain-sharing programs and described the conditions under which he believed such arrangements pose little risk to the Medicare program [7]. Also, under the Deficit Reduction Act of 2005, CMS is required to establish gain-sharing demonstrations to test methods and evaluate arrangements to improve quality and efficiency of care and hospital performance [8]. These comments by regulators and actions of legislators suggest the gain-sharing approach may be a more favorable and viable option in the future.

References

[1] Social Security Act § 1128B(b), 42 U.S.C.A. § 1320a-7b (2007).
[2] Social Security Act § 1877, 42 U.S.C.A. § 1395 (2007).
[3] Social Security Act § 1128A(b)(1)-(2), 42 U.S.C.A. § 1320a-7a (2007).
[4] Internal Revenue Code of 1986 § 501(c)(3), as amended, 26 U.S.C.A. § 501(c)(3) (2007).
[5] OIG Advisory Opinion No. 01-01.
[6] OIG Advisory Opinion No. 05-03.
[7] Hearings before Subcommittee on Health of the House Committee on Ways and Means. (October 7, 2005) (testimony of Lewis Morris, Chief Counsel to the Inspector General of the U.S. Department of Health and Human Services).
[8] Deficit Reduction Act of 2005, Pub. L. No. 109-171 § 5007(a), 120 Stat. 4, 34-36 (109th Cong. – 2nd Sess., Feb. 8, 2006).

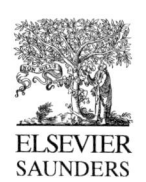

The Physician-Owned Imaging Center

Walter O'Neill, BS, R-PA

Orthopedic Imaging Partners, LLC, 7857 Noll Valley Road, Verona, WI 53593, USA

The advent of advanced imaging modalities in the past 20 years represents a paradigm shift as physicians seek new ways to offer earlier diagnosis and treatment and to augment practice service and revenues. This article elucidates this general trend in orthopedic imaging and examines practical aspects of the physician/practice-owned imaging center.

Imaging center history from an orthopedic perspective

Imaging in the form of conventional x-ray units has been a routine part of orthopedic practice since the late 1950s. Evaluating the quality of bone and fractures is one of the key clinical areas in orthopedics. In the case of trauma patients, typically the initial x-ray examination is performed in the hospital emergency room, with follow-up imaging via X ray done in the physician's office. Most nonemergency patients presenting to the orthopedic office have their initial x-ray evaluation done in the practice as well as follow-up examinations. As technology progressed from standard planar imaging with X ray to more computer-based imaging techniques (eg, CT) and nuclear medicine (bone scans), new tools were available for orthopedic physicians to evaluate patients with complex and infectious etiologies. As these new modalities were complex, expensive, and required dedicated rooms and dedicated staff, they were almost entirely purchased by hospital radiology departments and remained outside the direct ownership experience of most orthopedic practices.

In the early 1980s, the lifting of state and national regulations preventing non-hospital ownership of imaging equipment (certificate of need) presented new opportunities for entrepreneurial ownership of advanced imaging equipment. Early imaging centers were mostly local affairs, whereby a group of physicians, in conjunction with a local radiology group, formed a partnership to jointly own and operate imaging equipment outside the hospital. This came at a time when many hospitals were strapped for cash and unable to provide the necessary capital to purchase new equipment. Local physicians had access to capital and stepped into the opportunity to bring new technology to their communities via an imaging center. The trend took off with introduction of MRI technology, and many companies became national powerhouses, owning a 100 or more imaging centers by the late 1990s. These imaging centers often grew from a single modality to large centers that featured thousands of square feet offering a full range of imaging services, including CT, MRI, X ray, ultrasound, and nuclear medicine. In 1995, with the introduction of the Stark law restricting physician ownership in joint-venture projects, many orthopedic physicians were forced to divest ownership of the imaging centers in which they had been partners. The early experience of offering advanced imaging and the impact it had on patient management and surgical planning was not soon forgotten.

Advent of MRI

It was not until the advent of MRI systems, in the mid-1980s, that the promise of a new technique was realized that allows noninvasive visualization of soft-tissue structures of import to the orthopedic surgeon. The invention of early surface coils was critical to the development of techniques that allowed soft-tissue structures (ligaments, tendons, cartilage) inside the joint to

E-mail address: wjon3117@yahoo.com

be visualized with MRI. Early MRI studies of the knee by Crues and colleagues comparing results of knee arthroscopy to imaging had a powerful impact on both the radiology and orthopedic disciplines [1,2]. On the basis of this early evidence, other researchers built a variety of surface coils and conducted clinical studies to image other joints, including the shoulder, wrist, and hip. New collaborative efforts were undertaken by a group of dedicated musculoskeletal (MSK) radiologists and orthopedic surgeons to advance the clinical imaging science of imaging the joints. These efforts continue today.

The early 1990s saw a further refinement in MRI devices, with the extension of coil technology to phased-array and multichannel receiver systems, with the focus on delivering more signal-to-noise and higher-resolution images across all field strength units. The advent of open systems at this time was heavily marketed as an alternative to fixed cylindrical systems. Traditional cylindrical, high-field 1.5-T systems have evolved to today's "short-bore systems," which reduce the overall magnet size from an 8.5-ft magnet to 5 ft 4 in or shorter. This allows for the patient's upper body to be at the aperture of the magnet while undergoing a knee, foot, ankle, or lumbar spine study.

In the mid 1990s, a new imaging technology was introduced directly aimed at the orthopedic office: the extremity scanner (Fig. 1). The first scanners were small units with limited applications and low field and gradient strength. Their advantages included ease of siting (9 × 10 ft) room, low power requirements (110 V), no shielding requirements, and ease of use. Units such as the Artoscan, manufactured by Esaote and distributed in the United States by Lunar, were the first scanners that could be installed within a physician's office with a minimum of disruption to both the physical plant and staff (Fig. 2). Many orthopedic groups embraced this technology as a way to offer a new patient service, gain a competitive advantage, and augment practice revenue by capturing a revenue stream that they were previously referring to outside imaging centers or hospitals. As stated earlier, a large number of orthopedists already had prior ownership experience in an MRI through a local partnership before the Stark law. Ownership of an in-office MRI unit under the office ancillary exception under Stark became an attractive alternative to sending patients to the hospital or imaging center machines. From 1995 to 2000, the number of MRI units owned/operated by orthopedic groups grew from fewer than a dozen to several hundred.

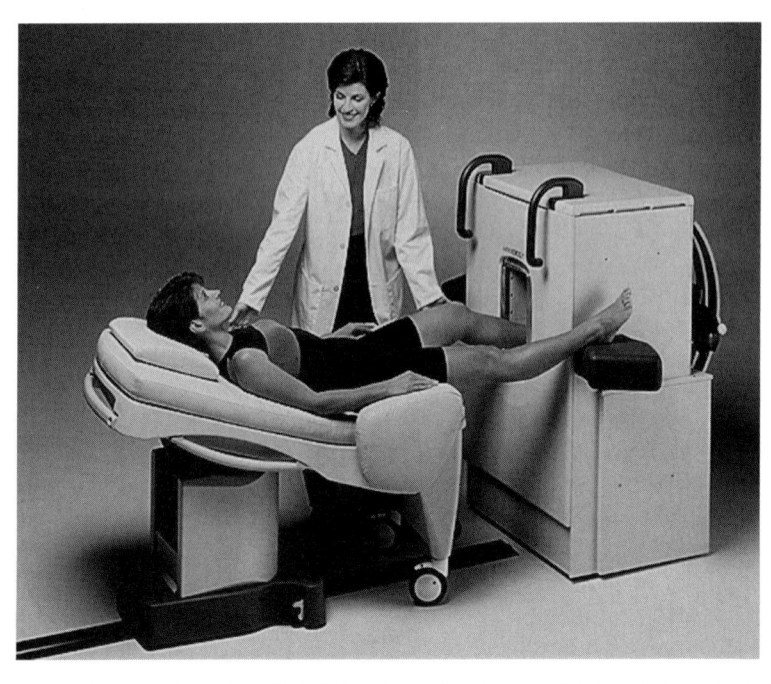

Fig. 1. The Artoscan system: the first extremity MRI system offered unparalleled patient comfort. (*Courtesy of* GE Healthcare; with permission.)

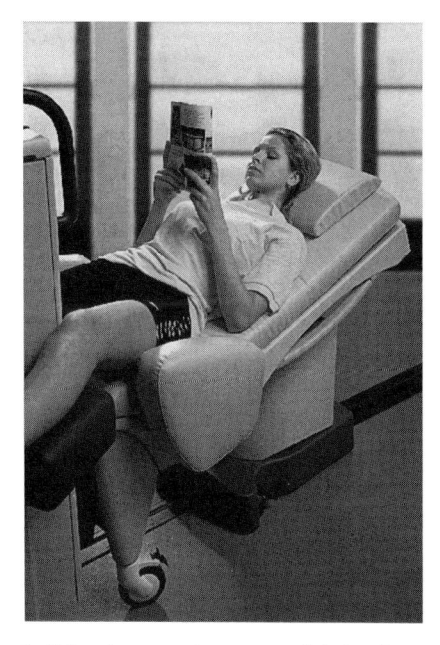

Fig. 2. Siting the extremity system minimizes impact on the office and staff. (*Courtesy of* GE Healthcare; with permission.)

New scanners from other companies have arrived in the market, including OrthoOne (ONI, Wilmington, MA), a high field strength (1.0 T) in an extremity MRI system (Fig. 3). At present, well over 800 practices offer MRI as a standard patient service.

When considering whole-body MRIs, more emphasis on the development of patient-friendly and lower-cost, permanent magnet-based systems has been the choice of many larger orthopedic groups (Fig. 4). These units offer lower operating and maintenance costs and the full breath of applications, including bilateral joint imaging and spine imaging. Similarly, costs of the traditional cylindrical, high field systems (Fig. 5) have been reduced approximately 20% to 25%, bringing them in the range of affordability of mid- to large-sized practices with a large percentage of patients requiring spine imaging. Aggressive leasing programs that couple the financing for the equipment and service as one monthly payment have made it even easier for most groups to acquire a unit of their own.

Developments in radiology have also played an important role in fostering the development of

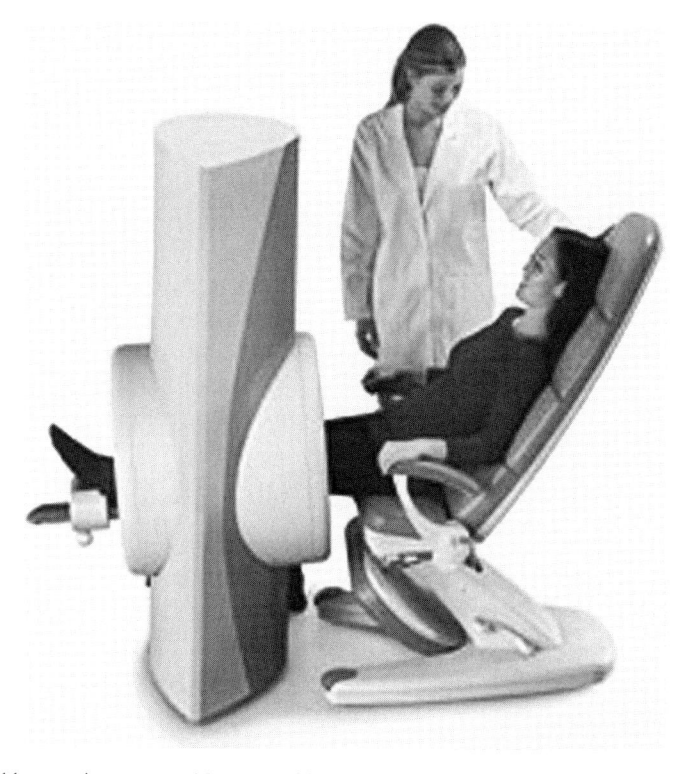

Fig. 3. ONI high field extremity scanner. (*Courtesy of* ONI Medical Systems, Inc., Wilmington, MA; with permission.)

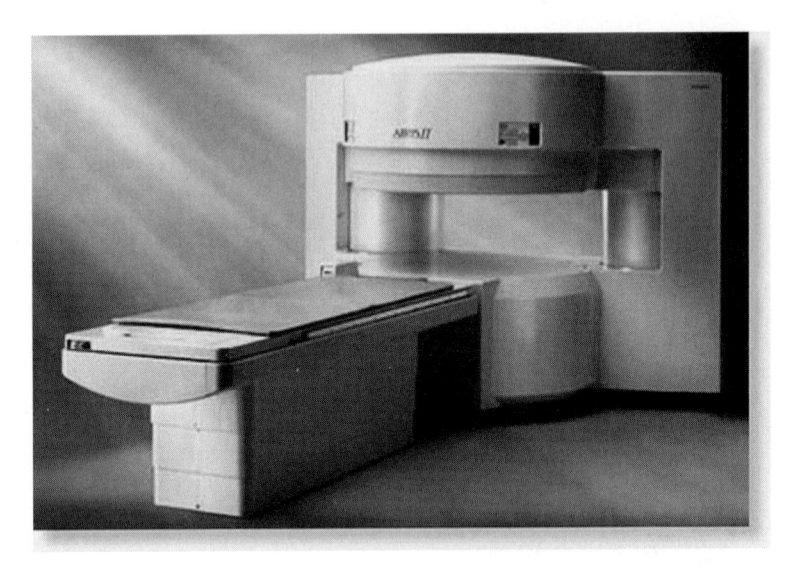

Fig. 4. Hitachi Airis system is an open, permanent magnet-based, whole-body scanner. (*Courtesy of* Hitchi America, Ltd, Brisbane, CA; with permission.)

office-based physician-owned imaging. MRI has matured in the last several years as protocols have become relatively fixed and imaging sequences established and refined. Coincident was the development of postgraduate fellowship programs in MSK radiology at a number of major universities in the United States. Most orthopedists were looking for on-line expertise to assist them with imaging interpretation of difficult cases, postsurgical imaging, and other imaging-related

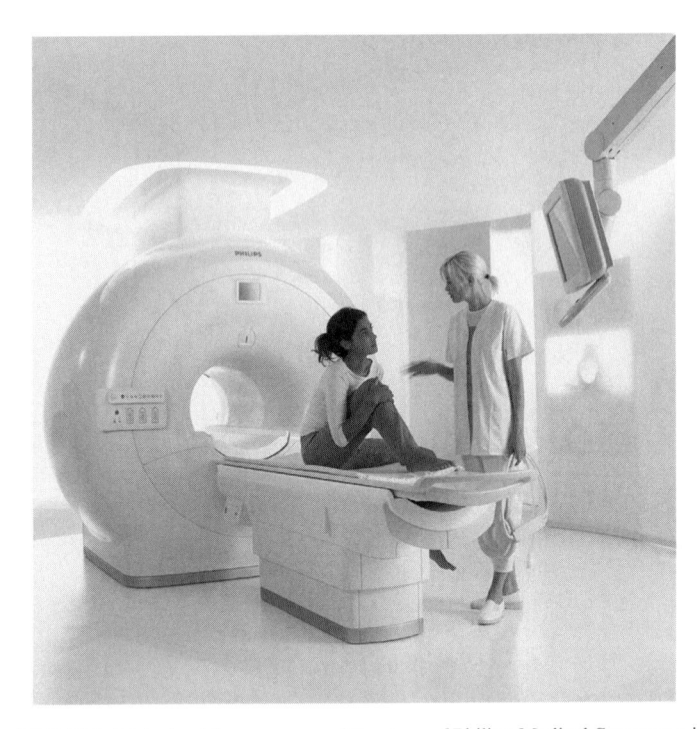

Fig. 5. Philips 1.5-T high field, short-bore scanner. (*Courtesy of* Philips Medical Systems; with permission.)

questions. Many were not pleased with the level of expertise in their local community. Practices of fellowship-trained MSK radiologists began marketing their on-line reading services via teleradiology to orthopedic groups that were purchasing an in-office extremity or whole-body unit (Fig. 6). This allowed the orthopedic groups to use imaging protocols created by MSK-specialized radiologists—imaging performed in their office by their staff whom the patients knew and trusted and the best interpretation by an MSK radiologist. This model today is the standard in orthopedics.

The physician-owned imaging center—update 2007

A physician-owned imaging center is defined as any imaging modality that is owned and operated by a physician or physician group. It may not be a freestanding imaging center that most people are familiar with, although some large groups have created multimodality centers that rival hospital and corporately owned centers. Physician-owned imaging in 2007 can include of a variety of modalities: X ray, computed radiography, digital radiography, ultrasound, bone mineral densitometry, CT and nuclear medicine, and picture archive and capture system in a myriad of settings. An extremity MRI scanner in a satellite office, whole-body MRI and CT units in a main facility, and another in a surgery center are just some examples. Digital x-ray systems tied into a picture archive and capture system for image distribution and review are another recent example. Just like the x-ray service that any orthopedic group routinely offers, physician-owned imaging can be used in a variety of settings and group situations. The reasons for embarking on a physician-owned imaging project and the revenues produced are as varied as the modalities they employ.

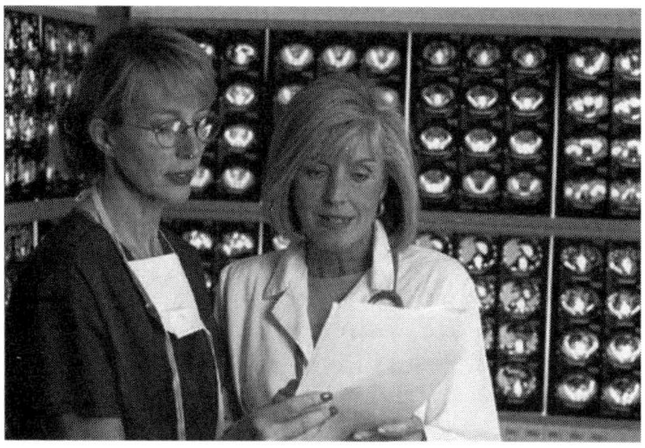

The discussion below explores the logic and considerations when undertaking a physician-owned imaging center project centered on MRI. Many of the siting, economic, and staffing considerations also apply to other modalities that may be considered by a growing practice.

The advantages of physician-owned imaging

Offering patients imaging services gives an office a competitive advantage by providing a wider variety of services from the patient's and the insurer's perspective. Some practices have used this approach to negotiate a single rate for everything, including a physical examination, X ray, MRI, surgery, and postsurgical care. There is evidence to suggest that those practices that offer in-house services are more efficient at returning patients to work quickly.

One of the major advantages of physician-owned in-office imaging is improved diagnostic accuracy. Orthopedic staff performs imaging examinations, with personalized protocols, interpreted by the radiologist of the orthopedist's choosing. This combination yields the best results for the patient, staff, and physician. Improved patient diagnosis via in-office imaging leads to more accurate surgery and faster recovery. Most practices have designated one or more of the x-ray technicians in the practice to operate the MRI unit and perform the studies in office (in the case of extremity MRI only, whole-body systems require a licensed MRI technician to operate). This gives the practice an economic advantage with little or no need to go outside to hire new staff. Many practices enlist the services of part-time x-ray technicians to perform the routine x-ray studies in the office while their full-time staff performs the MRIs. Assigning x-ray technicians to the MRI system is a significant growth opportunity for most employees and is an important tool to retain staff members who are critical to long-term success. In some cases, athletic trainers, physician extenders such as physician assistants, and nurse practitioners have performed MRI examinations. Some states require only licensed x-ray technicians, so it is important to verify the requirements in the particular state where the practice is located. Whole-body systems require licensed MRI technicians to operate the scanner, and many insurance companies are also requiring MRI technicians.

Fig. 6. With the advent of teleradiology, orthopedic surgeons can work with MSK radiologists of their choice ensuring more accurate imaging and interpretations.

Attracting new physicians to the practice has been a long-standing problem for many practices around the country. As more orthopedists reach retirement age, ancillary services such as MRI units can attract new physician talent to the practice. Often, practices that are located in rural areas or outside large metropolitan areas are at a disadvantage in hiring additional orthopedic surgeons. Adding an in-office MRI system is an added value to most physicians and considered a requirement by many fellowship-trained specialists accustomed to having an MRI located within their previous facilities with easy access and minimal patient waiting times.

Another advantage of an in-office MRI is that the patient remains within the group practice. A patient leaving the practice for outside studies may not return for follow-up or additional care. Retaining patients is an important aspect of practice management. In addition, if the group can avoid the phenomenon know as "satellite patients" (ie, where patients leave the practice and "revolve around it" while having their imaging studies performed, interpreted, filmed, and collated before returning), patients can easily be scheduled for surgery if indicated.

Many publications have cited the economic rewards of owning and operating an in-office MRI unit. However, there are also benefits provided to the community when adding MRI to the group practice. It allows the physician to offer the MRI service to indigent athletes and other patients who otherwise would not be able to afford to have these studies performed. A number of practices have also performed scans on patients at little or no charge to monitor healing rates of new surgical procedures. Many National Football League team physicians have used scanners to evaluate professional athletes to certify injury healing before training camps and after injuries in weekly games. In a few cases, colleges have contracted with orthopedic groups that offer MRI services so that while they manage the college athlete's physical care, they also perform the MRIs on the student athletes.

Comparison of physician-owned imaging with outside imaging

Several people have suggested that the studies done in a physician-owned scanner are less accurate or less diagnostic than those performed in an hospital or freestanding imaging center controlled by a radiologist. Anecdotal and published literature repudiates that assertion.

Several studies have been published that favorably compare the results from in-office units with results from high field units and arthroscopy [3]. Having an extremity or in-office scanner is not the only issue in rendering a useful diagnosis. A highly skilled magnetic resonance operator is critical as well. An in-office scanner with preprogrammed protocols operated by a skilled operator and supervised by an orthopedic group with an experienced MSK radiologist performing the interpretations represents the highest level of MSK imaging.

Experience indicates that imaging times on an extremity scanner are comparable to scan times on whole-body units. Typical scan times range from 26 to 32 minutes for the knee or shoulder, respectively. The imaging capability of an extremity scanner in terms of sensitivity and specificity has been favorably compared both to high field units and arthroscopy [3]. Scan resolution and image field of view are comparable to those produced on imaging-center or hospital-based units. Whole-body units used by orthopedic groups have the full complement of imaging sequences used by imaging centers or hospitals and are completely comparable. Most recently, the American College of Radiology has required that full-body MRI sites pass a series of tests to achieve certification of site status by the College. Some insurance providers have used this point as a differentiator when choosing sites to reimburse for MRI studies performed in office. Similar criteria are being established for extremity systems as well with the main accrediting body, the Intersocietal Commission for the Accreditation of Magnetic Resonance Laboratories, offering the certification. Certainly it is prudent for any orthopedic site to seek accreditation.

Evaluating physician-office MRI choices

It is important to provide a framework to enable the orthopedic physician to make critical decisions regarding the myriad of choices of systems that are on the market. The appropriate MRI unit can be selected based on clinical applicability, acquisition cost, and operating costs (Box 1).

The first key factor when looking at any imaging decision is to understand clearly the number of patients that the practice generates

> **Box 1. Key factors that influence the decision to acquire an MRI**
>
> - Patient volume
> - Anatomic distribution of exams (spines versus extremities)
> - Image quality
> - Payer mix
> - Siting (space to locate magnet)
> - Financing
> - Physician preferences (perception of open versus closed)
> - Prior MRI experience
> - Local political climate (hospital relationship)
> - Radiologist preferences and relationships
> - Other plans for expansion (ambulatory surgery center, etc)

who can be imaged on the practice-owned MRI unit. These patient-volume data and a payer analysis will be used to determine the amount of revenue generated for the group practice. In the case of MRI, it is critical that the data that are used to make the decision be of the highest quality possible. Anecdotal information such as, "I was in the office yesterday and referred out seven MRI studies" is useless when making such a critical economic decision. A formal survey of patient referrals by each physician typically collected for 30 days by that physician's scheduler is critical. For groups smaller than five physicians, 45 days or more of data may be required, as vacations or attendance at off-site meetings may result in an incomplete database when collections are shorter than 1 month. In areas of the country that depend on seasonal variations in patient volume (eg, Florida, the Gulf Coast, Arizona, and certain areas in the mountains close to ski areas), other analysis may be required to balance data.

Along with the volume of patient studies that the practice is generating, it is critical to determine which body areas are most frequently being scanned. One of the key decisions a practice needs to make as to whether to select a whole-body scanner versus an extremity scanner clearly depends on the volume of spine scans. As extremity magnets are made such that the magnet needs to magnetize only the limb that is introduced into the magnetic field, they are by design less costly to build than whole-body systems. Moreover, 50% of the cost an MRI system is the magnet itself, so selecting the right scanner based on the clinical applications planned to be imaged can make the difference economically for the group, with a significant variance in return on investment.

Image quality is of paramount import when making a decision on adding an office MRI to one's practice. Considerations of MRI image quality, however, are not necessarily straightforward. Although field strength used to be the main determinant of image quality, developments in coil technology have seen systems at low-field (<0.3 T) and midfield strength (0.35–0.5 T) producing images that are comparable to high field systems. MRI has the unique property that, while it uses non-ionizing radiation, the same information can be acquired and summed to yield better images (signal averaging). Although making an MRI image is a function of the equipment (ie, field strength, magnetic homogeneity, coil technology, slice thickness, resolution, postprocessing algorithms, etc), the operator, and patient geometry, it involves a number of technical tradeoffs. If time is not a primary limitation— patients will normally tolerate most examinations that take no more than 40–45 minutes—signal-averaging techniques can be used to improve image quality. When evaluating images that are produced on the machine that is under consideration, weigh the resolution (detail) and conspicuity of the anatomy of interest. Is it easy to see the structures of primary interest? Can the decision to plan surgery be based confidently on what can be discerned in the viewed images? What was the length of the examination? Is the time something that fits in well with the practice's plan of patient volume and staffing? These are a few of the questions that must be answered before moving forward.

As the myriad choices of machine are evaluated, there are some ways to ensure that the images provided by the various vendors are representative of what a machine will produce at the actual facility. Requesting images that reflect an entire case provides a more complete picture of how all the sequences image the patient anatomy in question. Make sure to note the techniques used and scan times if possible; ask for a list of references that have the same scanner of interest and call the physicians at that site. Are they happy with the overall operation of the machine? Is the image quality what they expected? Are they performing all studies on the unit, or are members of the group sending patients for outside MRIs? If possible, ask them to have their technicians pick a couple of random cases, double film them, and send a set. If there is time, visit a site to see the equipment in question in operation. Take a member of the group as a volunteer and request the images after his or her examination. This is an easy way to reassure the other member of the practice that the right decision can be made.

Payer issues are among some of the most difficult challenges facing an orthopedic practice. This also applies to in-office, physician-owned imaging. A general rule of thumb is that if a particular insurance company is currently reimbursing a practice for performing surgery, it is likely that it will also reimburse for imaging. Although this is a general rule, there are exceptions across the country. When assembling the data during the feasibility part of the project, it is important to list each payer next to the patient anatomy scanned and the appropriate *Current Procedural Terminology* (*CPT*) code, which can be obtained from the CPT code book or most MRI vendors (Table 1). Office staff should take the CPT codes, collate them, and request the payment schedule from the insurance company. This analysis will yield the subset of all the MRI studies that could be performed for which an office will actually get reimbursed and will provide the final revenue figures for the feasibility study.

Siting an in-office MRI system

Siting a magnet in an orthopedic practice is often a challenge. Most practices do not have a room already designated as the MRI suite. Siting of extremity versus whole-body systems due to their different requirements can be difficult. There are a few general rules regarding the placement of the MRI system and the surrounding environment. Preferred placement of an MRI system includes sites on the first floor of a building (slab on grade) and away from elevators, transformers, and moving metal (such as cars, trucks, buses) and not over a parking garage. These hazards can often be overcome with special shielding or compensation circuitry at a significant additional cost.

In most cases, siting an extremity magnet is a relatively easy and not particularly costly proposition. Typically, an extremity system can be sited in a space as small as 100 ft^2 (C-Scan) or a room that is 14 × 17 ft for a shoulder-based extremity MRI unit. The average cost of demolition of the space and renovation is in the range of $15,000 to $18,000. Obviously, if the system is sited in a building where there are structural issues, costs could run higher. Subdividing a cast room to accommodate an MRI, or moving one wall of an examination room a few feet, can create spaces of this size. Extremity MRI units do not require special electrical requirements, but rather use a dedicated 110-V 20-A outlet. In addition, they often do not require the added cost of a dedicated air conditioner, provided there is adequate cooling and heating in the space and the building's heating, ventilation, and air conditioning system stays activated overnight.

Delivery of an extremity MRI system is usually straightforward. The largest single piece of the MRI system is the magnet, and it is designed to roll through a standard doorway and hallways into the final resting space through portals of as small as 33 in.

MRI vendors typically include the cost of the radio-frequency (RF) screening (shielding) in their price quotes to customers. RF shielding is required to screen out extraneous radio waves from entering the MRI room that would overwhelm the sensitive receive channels of the MRI system and adversely affect image quality. This saves a practice about $30,000 to $45,000 and has the added advantage of having the vendor coordinate the shielding installation and folding the maintenance (warranty) for the shielding into the vendor's service contract. There are really two choices for RF enclosures for an extremity MRI unit: a freestanding RF pavilion (most suited to open sites like a physical therapy space) and the standard RF room (particularly good for smaller spaces). The choice of which one is most appropriate is

Table 1
Current procedural terminology codes for MRI of the extremities

Anatomy	No contrast	With contrast	With and without
MRI of upper extremity	73 218	73 219	73 220
MRI of joint of upper extremity	73 221	73 222	73 223
MRI of lower extremity	73 718	73 719	73 720
MRI of joint of lower extremity	73 721	73 722	73 723

often governed by the geometry and space available within the office.

For whole-body systems, siting is a more complicated and costly project. Decisions on siting, power, and layout are best left to professional architects, structural engineers, and installation specialists from the MRI manufacturers. These professionals can accumulate the data regarding the site specifics and preferred magnets, and present the practice management staff with site recommendations for review.

Depending on the magnet selected (open versus closed), the siting of the systems needs to also encompass containment of the magnetic field as well as structural issues. Typical whole-body magnets require a suite size of approximately 500 to 700 ft^2 arranged in three rooms: the largest is for the magnet (typically 16 × 24 ft), one is for the electronics, and the third for the operator's console. Siting a whole-body magnet is significantly easier and less costly on a first-floor slab on grade site. When installing permanent magnet systems, weight considerations (magnet of 40,000 lb or more) make the first floor the least costly and most practical solution.

All whole-body systems have specific power requirements that need to be taken into consideration. These power requirements vary from 208/220 to 480 V power and require additional transfers to step up power that is available in most buildings. Prudence and code mandate that a local electrician, in conjunction with the vendor's installation and planning specialists, approve the electrical distribution in the MRI suite.

Most MRI vendors require the practice to pay for the final delivery of the system via either movers or professional riggers. This is an important consideration, and in the case of whole-body systems, not a trivial cost for the group to consider. For extremity systems, such costs are in the range of $1500 to $5000. For whole-body systems, the costs can range from $10,000 to as high as $50,000 for complicated deliveries using a crane in a multistory building.

The role of financing for a physician-owned imaging project

Financing is a key component of making the final decision regarding the feasibility; ultimately, it has a direct effect on the profitability of an MRI project for the practice. Financing obviates the need for the group to come up with the full purchase price of the scanner at the beginning of the project, or to make "progress payments" as most vendor contracts specify, even though the system is not fully installed or in use. Leasing in essence allows the practice to "cash flow" the acquisition of the scanner by using funds received for scans performed to pay the lease and expense of the project. It also allows a group to use financing expense to offset the revenue produced to minimize tax exposure. It is wise to accrue several months of operating expenses when starting a project owing to the start-up costs (marketing, staffing, site improvements, etc) while balancing the account receivables that will be negative until the first payments are received (typically 60–90 days after the scans are performed). Many of these costs can be reduced by vendor-leasing programs that offer financing for "soft costs" such as new furniture, lease-hold improvements, and skip payments all rolled into a single package. Choosing the right financing package to suit the group's needs is a decision that is best made with the group's accountants/financial advisers involved.

Orthopedic groups have several choices for financing. Bank financing is always an available source of funds to purchase the MRI unit. Although banks like to provide capital for building projects such as an ASC, they often lack the prowess on high-technology items and often use extremely conservative estimates when calculating residual values on fair market value leases, which yield higher monthly payments for the practice. In addition, banks do not have an expertise on the disposal/removal of the equipment at the end of the lease and cannot offer popular programs where service is rolled into the lease and paid monthly along with the equipment. Leasing through the vendor's leasing programs is a popular choice for most practices considering a physician-owned imaging project. Leasing via vendor leasing companies with a vendor-supported fair market value lease has the added advantage of low capital cost, up-front costs, and no progress fees. The typical lease requires one monthly lease payment initially, and then the payments begin once the unit begins operation. This allows the practice to build up receivables before having to make the lease payments and ensures that cash flow for the practice is preserved. Leasing and financing terms should be chosen that match the terms of the project. The group strategy should be to match the time of use of the equipment in the practice with the lease term. If the group knows that a new building is to be constructed in 3 years, a 36-month lease would be the best choice. In the case of a solo practice with an emphasis on the lowest monthly payments, extending the payment terms from the standard 60 months to 72 or even 84 months makes sense. Working with the practice's administrator, vendor sales consultant, and accountant is the best way to customize a leasing program that is best for each practice.

The physician-owned imaging project: other considerations

Physician experience and preference are important factors that influence the choice of MRI unit to purchase. Some physicians prefer the ability to perform spine scans on closed systems, whereas others prefer to scan all patients on open systems. Prior experience with other MRI systems in a community often prejudices physicians on which system to choose. This may not be a fair representation of what the unit is capable of and should not be the basis of an orthopedic group's evaluation without further investigation. The outcome of the right MRI decision for an orthopedic group is that each member is satisfied that the scanner selected can answer their specific clinical questions, accommodate their patient population, and do so while bringing revenue to the practice.

The local political environment is a secondary consideration when considering the feasibility of an MRI project for the group. Hospitals and radiology groups can be quite threatened when confronted with an orthopedic group that has informed them that an imaging project is imminent. It is important that any orthopedic group planning to add an MRI or other imaging to the office consider these reactions in advance and create plans for dealing with them. It is critical for the group to also clearly understand any constraints via real estate lease exclusions before embarking on an imaging project. If the practice is located in a medical outpatient building owned by the hospital, it is of paramount importance to know whether the lease excludes imaging facilities per se. This can be hidden in a clause that states something ambiguous such as, "XYZ Orthopedic group agrees that while of a tenant of ZZZ building that it not compete with any hospital services without the express written consent of the hospital board of directors." In all cases, it is wise to have the group's attorney review the office lease before embarking on any imaging project.

Radiologists who are friendly and supportive of an orthopedic group make great allies. They can provide guidance and be critical in the evaluation of systems, especially when it comes to whole-body systems. Having a trusted radiologist is also critical to the success of the in-office project. It is recommended that the orthopedic group retain the services of a fellowship-trained MSK radiologist when considering possible readers for the office-based project. Although many orthopedic physicians feel comfortable with performing their own interpretations of the MRI images, the standard of care for the country is to have a radiologist perform the official interpretation. Using local radiologists is a good move politically; however, it may not be such a good move if the reading expertise of the group in town is not sufficient to support the specialized MRI project. To fill this void, there are a number of teleradiology services that offer fellowship-trained MSK radiologists (licensed in most states) on line to provide interpretations.

Last among the considerations for a group to consider is to compare the priority of the in-office imaging project with that of all of the other projects the group may be embarking on. One also needs to consider, in the context of return on investment and competitive advantage, whether other projects (like an ASC) that use the practice's capital and earning power would be a better investment in the near term.

The economic story of a physician-owned imaging project

The economics of in-office imaging are relatively easy to understand. There are the fixed costs of the lease, financing of the unit, service expense, and the overhead costs of the site. One should include in the overhead figure the salaries and benefits of the technologists who are assigned to the MRI unit and the space it uses in the office. There are some variable costs, which include utilities such as electricity, consumables such as shorts that the patients will wear, and storage media for the images (whether film or electronic). If technicians are paid by the hour for any overtime or weekend work, that will be an additional variable cost. Any time revenue exceeds these costs, the practice is generating a profit.

A simplified financial equation for an in-office imaging project is as follows:

Revenues (patient volume
  × payer reimbursement)
  − Expenses (lease, technicians,
    service, overhead, etc) = Gross profit

The goal of a particular project should be determined by the members of the group. Some groups have philosophical discussions to determine the relative importance of profit optimization versus offering a patient service and balancing the political climate in their location. In some instances, groups will choose the solution that offers the most complete patient service (extremity versus whole body), based on their patient volume and breadth of their clinical practice while offering the group a reasonable return on their investment.

In the author's actual experience, patient volume naturally increases about 10% to 15% in the first year, owing to the convenience factor of having the scanner within the practice. The increase in patient volume is something that has been demonstrated in most MRI projects across the country, whether in orthopedic offices or in freestanding centers. Although not a major factor in the pro forma, it is one that should be considered but not necessarily included in the initial plan.

Another factor that the orthopedic group should determine is its gross break-even point. It can be easily calculated by inserting actual values in the following equation:

Monthly expenses/Average reimbursement/
  20 working-days month
  = Breakeven in patients per day

The number generated by the break-even calculation is an important determinant of the likelihood of financial success, given the dynamics of the group's particular market (reimbursement levels, technician salaries, etc). It is also essential when examining the economics of one MRI system versus another (ie, extremity versus whole body). Most MRI vendors will communicate the economic advantages of their offerings by the use of a break-even analysis. As an example, most extremity systems are in the range of 1.2 to 1.4 patients per day to break even. Whole-body projects typically start in the range of 3 to 4 patients per day, given their higher build-out costs and price of the equipment; the break-even point for more complex and costly projects can range upwards of 6 to 7 patients per day. As mentioned above, matching patient volume (revenue) is critical for achieving success of an in-office imaging project success.

Economic discussion of other modalities

Other modalities such as CT, ultrasound, and nuclear cameras essentially follow the same line of reasoning and economic justification that was presented here for MRI. Patient volume and clinical application appropriateness are just a few of the key factors involved. With ultrasound, siting is really not an issue as most ultrasound machines are relatively compact and can be wheeled from office to office as needed. In many cases with ultrasound, the physician is performing the studies directly, which obviously involves direct time investment and training on the part of the physician. CT is used by some practices for specific views of the spine and to plan patient surgery and management with complex three-dimensional fractures as well as certain new implants. CT prices have come down in the last several years, and many multislice models are available from original equipment manufacturer vendors at low prices. Reimbursement for CT examinations is approximately 60% of MRI examinations, with the same breakout between technical and professional charges. A CT scanner may be sited in a room that is 14 × 16 ft and requires lead shielding and special power. Break-even points on a CT can run from 2 to 3 patients per day once staffing and space requirements are figured into the pro forma. As in all cases, it is best to check with the vendor for its financial projections and to check them against the practice's own forecasts.

Computed radiography and digital radiography systems (which replace conventional x-ray technology) feature more complicated financial pro formas, which include consideration for the replacement of film costs, chemistry, reclamation of dark room space, reduction/elimination of film storage, and possible reduction of staff needed to take and file X rays. These variables are outside the scope of this article, but should be factored in by every practice that is considering building a new office, replacing older x-ray equipment, or moving its facility.

Summary

A physician-owned, office-based imaging project has evolved from conventional x-ray to more advanced imaging, which includes MRI, CT, and other digital imaging methods. Orthopedic practices need to do a thorough analysis to match the technology and type of unit to their patient volume and prospective payment for the services rendered. This analysis should include understanding the capability and limitations of the MRI or other imaging modality selected, staffing, siting, and teleradiology interpretations. Only after such analysis can the practice be assured of a successful project.

References

[1] Crues JV, Ryu R, Morgan FW. Meniscal pathology: the expanding role of MRI. Clin Orthop 1990;252:80–7.
[2] Crues JV III, Mink, Levy TL, et al. Meniscal tears of the knee: accuracy of MR imaging. Radiology 1987;164:445–8.
[3] Shellock F, Bert J, Fritts H, et al. Evaluation of the rotator cuff and glenoid labrum using a .2 Tesla dedicated extremity MR system: MR results compared to surgical findings. Radiology 2003;221:435–48.

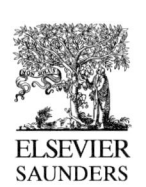

The Physician-Owned Physical Therapy Department
Paul Duxbury, PT, ATC/R
1560 Beam Avenue, Suite D, Maplewood, MN 55109, USA

Access to high-quality physical therapy care is just as important to patients as access to high-quality diagnostic and surgical facilities to maximize their functional outcomes in a timely fashion.

Internalization of physical therapy services within the clinic as either an off-site or on-site entity offers the opportunity to assure patient access to the highest quality of rehabilitation services under the group's supervision and direction. The internalized physical therapy department offers a number of advantages over an independent, external provider that are likely to improve services and outcomes for orthopedic patients. Continuity of care is enhanced by the convenience of scheduling of physical therapy services. The patient is much more likely to follow through with the physician's physical therapy wishes because, with a centralized scheduling system, the patient will have the opportunity to schedule appointments immediately upon receiving physical therapy orders. Alternately, the patient can walk down the hall to schedule an appointment and possibly be seen immediately.

Another direct advantage to patients receiving physician-owned physical therapy services is the ease of access the therapist will have to the patient's medical record. Unimpaired access to pertinent medical records including diagnostic tests, operative reports, and physician examination notes will give the treating physical therapist a significant advantage in understanding and addressing patient's needs in a timely fashion. The time needed to exchange this valuable information with an independent provider could easily delay positive interventions for several days or more.

Furthermore, if the group is less than satisfied with the current physical therapy provider(s), the internalization of physical therapy services allows the hiring of staff with the attributes the group desires and the ability to provide the staff with incentives to ensure the delivery of the highest possible quality of care.

As the trend toward shrinking reimbursement for physician services continues, an internal physical therapy clinic providing high-quality care and a source of additional revenue presents an attractive opportunity.

A variety of physician practice specialties might consider internalizing outpatient physical therapy services. Orthopedic, neurosurgery, occupational health, and relatively large family practice groups are the practices that have the potential to generate the volume of physical therapy referrals that would make internalization of these services practical from a financial perspective. Orthopedic surgery is the physician specialty that most commonly internalizes physical therapy successfully.

Once the decision has been made to investigate seriously the possibility of an internal physical therapy practice, a number of issues need to be explored and questions answered. It then becomes important to have experienced individuals address legal and local physical therapy issues. These issues include Medicare compliance, reimbursement, referral patterns, competition, and contracting as well as the development of a successful business plan.

Keys to success are the development of an accurate financial pro-forma analysis and group decisions involving location, space planning, and staffing. The first challenge is to ascertain whether the practice will generate adequate physical therapy referral volumes to make an internal physical therapy clinic viable. Successful planning for the

E-mail address: pduxbury@summitortho.com

clinic will depend on the group's ability to predict accurately the volume of physical therapy referrals generated by the group physicians and the resulting number of physical therapy visits resulting from those referrals that ultimately receive care at the physical therapy clinic.

Facility space needs and staffing requirements are dictated by the anticipated number of patient visits. There is no simple formula for determining this number. There are wide variations in physical therapy referral patterns both between and within physician specialties.

The most accurate method of predicting group referral volumes is to track the current external physical therapy referrals for a period of time. The longer the tracking period, the more accurate the prediction will be. The group must be sensitive to geographic concerns and include only physical therapy referrals in which the patient would be compliant in attending multiple physical therapy visits at the proposed site. One way to accomplish this would be to include referrals of patients who have a work or home address with a zip code within a reasonable commuting distance and time from the physical therapy clinic. The group also must research what, if any, restrictions from a payer or closed network may impact the referral pattern.

Once the group determines the average number of referrals per physician, the next step is to determine the average number of visits per referral. These two variables allow calculation of the projected annual physical therapy visits, the key statistic needed to determine space and staffing needs. The average number of patient visits per physical therapy referral can vary widely between physicians for a variety of reasons, including physician specialty (eg, occupational health physicians versus orthopedic surgeons), philosophy of care, and personal experience. A simple method of obtaining this statistic is to review physical therapy discharge summaries of patients from the referring physicians; these summaries frequently include the patient's total number of visits. Another source of this information may be the physical therapist(s) who treat patients from the practice. Other possible sources of these data might include a local physical therapist who is being recruited, a health care consultant, or a payer representative.

In most situations one should expect that 90% to 95% of the patient referral volumes will be generated internally. Exceptions to this rule, such as the recruitment of a physical therapist with a loyal referral base and/or patient following (ie, a physical therapist with expertise in treating chronic pain or throwing athletes) or an unfulfilled need for physical therapy services in the geographic area, must be considered. One must be sure to include the anticipated growth of the group physician practice into the physical therapy projections.

Financial projections for the physical therapy department will be driven by projected annual patient visits. On the expense side, patient visits will dictate staffing and space needs. Staff salaries and rent constitute approximately 80% to 90% of annual expenses. Other significant expenses include supplies, information technology, and administrative services. Staffing expenses are influenced by the particular staffing model the group finds most useful. Staffing models and other related issues are discussed later in this article.

An experienced physical therapist or physical therapist assistant could be expected to treat around 2500 to 2800 patients per calendar year, at a rate of 50 to 55 patients per week. This estimate assumes a 40-hour workweek, 1-hour initial visits with half-hour repeat visits, and a schedule cancellation rate of 10%. For example, staffing needs for 10,000 annual patient visits would include four providers, a receptionist and/or scheduler, and the appropriate business office and administrative support.

Reliable revenue projections for the physical therapy department probably will require knowledge of local payer-specific reimbursement data. This information, combined with the projected payer mix and annual patient visits, should allow a fairly accurate calculation of expected revenues.

Capital expenses are relatively reasonable in the initial phase of development of the physical therapy business venture. Routine physical therapy–specific equipment needs include modalities such as ultrasound, electrical stimulation, mechanical traction machine, iontophoresor, a hydrocollator unit, and treatment tables. Exercise equipment is important and necessary in an active rehabilitation environment. Capital needs in this area include treadmill(s), stationary exercise cycle(s), stair stepper(s) (upright and/or recumbent), and leg press, leg extension, and leg curl machines. Less elaborate equipment needs include stabilization balls, free weights, and balance systems.

In addition to this equipment, other optional high-tech pieces of equipment could easily double or triple the initial capital equipment expenses. An example is an isokinetic exercise machine that can be used for evaluation purposes as well as rehabilitation. This type of equipment would not be a necessity for a start-up or general practice physical therapy clinic but might add value to a clinic desiring a specific niche. A physical therapy clinic targeting the occupational health market may benefit from isokinetic equipment test results that can be used to validate return-to-work status and identify potential malingerers. This type of equipment also is an impressive marketing tool to employers and others involved in returning injured employees to work in a safe and timely manner. Isokinetic equipment also can add value to the sports physical therapy clinic to rehabilitate and monitor the progress of athletes and aid in the return-to-sport decision-making process. The lead physical therapist can provide guidance about rehabilitative equipment priorities. Patient profiles and treatment philosophy will influence equipment needs. Last, it is important to budget for office equipment (ie, copier, fax machine, furniture, and information technology).

One of the major decisions to be determined is where to locate the internal physical therapy clinic. Until 1999, physician-owned physical therapy services had to be provided on site. "On site" was defined as a physician clinic in which two or more physicians practiced medicine. At least one physician had to be on site during all hours of clinic operation, and physical therapy services had to be billed incident to physician services. In 1999 the Center for Medicare and Medicaid Services (CMS) allowed physician-employed physical therapists to practice off site, billing for services with their own provider identification numbers (PIN). This legislation provided physicians more flexibility in the delivery of physical therapy services. Physicians now are allowed to consider locations off site from the physician's clinic to provide physical therapy services. A single physician group now can have multiple internal physical therapy clinics. A discussion of the CMS requirement for off-site versus on-site physical therapy is beyond the scope of this article except to note that physical therapists practicing off-site must have their own PINs. It is imperative to obtain advice from a health care attorney concerning CMS requirements that pertain to physician-owned physical therapy services.

There are other issues to consider when determining the location of the internal physical therapy clinic. The advantages of the on-site location include "walkover" referrals that allow patients to schedule their physical therapy appointments and possibly be seen immediately if the physical therapist's schedule permits. The convenience and familiarity offered to the patient in this setting contributes to the likelihood that the patient will follow through with the physical therapy orders. The efficiency of the physical therapist also is enhanced in this setting because of the increased potential of a walk-in patient's filling open slots in the schedule. Another advantage of the on-site clinic is that of "corridor consultations," in which the physical therapists and physicians can consult with one another on the spur of the moment to address the patient's needs in a timely fashion.

Key advantages to the off-site physical therapy clinic include the opportunity to seek out space that is more accessible to the clinic patients while possibly decreasing the cost of medical office space. Addressing accessibility issues for the patients, especially parking, will increase patient compliance with physical therapy orders and improve clinic productivity.

Possibly the most important decision the group will make in determining the overall quality of service provided by the physical therapy clinic is the selection of the lead physical therapist. This individual should be an experienced, respected professional with proven leadership and clinical skills. It is critical to assess this individual's attitude and personality, because this therapist will set the tone for the entire clinic. This person will be responsible for motivating staff to meet and exceed the patients' physical therapy expectations. The performance of the lead therapist obviously will influence the patient's opinion of the physician's decision to refer him or her to the physical therapy clinic. Ideally, this the lead therapist will have an existing referral relationship with one or more of the group's physicians. He or she may be the therapist to whom the physicians refer their difficult patients. Initially, this individual may serve in a consulting capacity during the planning and development stages. This therapist should be an excellent source for information on pertinent physical therapy issues, reimbursement trends, staffing models, and productivity expectations.

The next decision will be to decide on a specific staffing model. A variety of staffing models exist in physical therapy clinics, with various combinations of physical therapists, physical therapist assistants (PTAs), physical therapy aides, and certified athletic trainers. The staffing model best suited for the clinic's needs depends on a number of factors. First, the staffing model will be determined by CMS, state, and payor rules and regulations that pertain to the provision and billing of physical therapy services. Legal counsel and the lead physical therapist should be consulted regarding these issues.

If the practice sees a varied mix of patient types, the group should consider physical therapists who have a general orthopedic background and an area of interest or expertise such as golf, swimming, or specialized manual therapy skills. The physical therapist will be responsible for the initial evaluation of the patient and determining the care plan. The physical therapist may be supported by a PTA and/or a physical therapy aide. A PTA is best used in a setting where a relatively high percentage of extremity, rather than spine, patients are seen. PTAs are not as well utilized in settings where a relatively high percentage of spine or Medicare patients are seen. Spine patients routinely receive manual treatment techniques for which PTAs lack training or that are beyond their scope of practice. Medicare supervision requirements for PTAs can be burdensome to the supervising physical therapist.

Physical therapy aides are used primarily for rooming patients, treatment set-ups, and cleaning/laundry duties. They generally are not permitted to take an active role in the treatment or supervision of the physical therapy patient.

The role of the certified athletic trainer (ATC) in the physical therapy clinic is regulated and varies from state to state. The ATC may serve a potentially beneficial role marketing clinic services to local high schools or athletic clubs. Responsibilities may include serving as an athletic trainer for games and/or practices and as an evaluator of athletic injuries on or off site.

When the group is hiring physical therapists, it should seek to create a staff with diverse areas of expertise. Therapists who have personal experience in a particular sport or specialized training in a niche area offer an advantage over the competition and create an opportunity to attract additional external referrals.

Another key to success is the proper space design for the clinic. Successful space design will benefit from the services of an experienced outpatient physical therapist and a space designer with a background in health care projects. Collaboration between the lead physical therapist and the space designer probably will yield the best overall design.

Space design should be addressed after volume projections have been completed. Considerations include the number and size of the treatment rooms, the size of the gym area, reception area, waiting room, staff office, laundry facilities, and storage space for supplies and modalities. Space dedicated to a whirlpool room is not a necessity for most clinics. Use and reimbursement may not justify inclusion of a whirlpool area in the clinic.

A successful space design will create an atmosphere that is professional and appealing. It will provide unobstructed patient flow and patient privacy. The appearance of the physical therapy practice will contribute to patients' overall assessment of the medical practice. The professional image portrayed in the practice should carry over to the physical therapy facilities. The positive impression patients get as they enter the physical therapy clinic for the first time will confirm their confidence in the physician's judgment and in the care they will receive.

The lead physical therapist will play a significant role in determining the philosophy of care practiced by the clinic staff. The physical therapy care provided at the facility should be tailored to each patient's individual needs. A thorough evaluation performed at the time of the initial visit should identify injury-related objective and functional limitations. The physical therapist will use these findings to establish a set of time-specific functional goals. Included in these goals should be the patient's ability to self-manage the condition and be independent in a home exercise program.

Active care including therapeutic exercise, education, and manual therapy often is recommended over passive modalities such as hot packs, ultrasound, and massage. This approach to therapy encourages patients to have an active role in their rehabilitation programs.

Manual therapy is defined as specific hands-on techniques, including manipulation and mobilization, to diagnose and treat soft tissue injuries and joint structures. Examples of manual therapy include mobilization of the spine and extremities, myofascial release, and muscle energy techniques. Manual therapy has proven effective in managing both acute and chronic musculoskeletal conditions. Therapeutic exercise includes strengthening, endurance, and range-of-motion activities intended to assist the patient in overcoming functional deficits. Passive modalities can be effective as an adjunct to an active rehabilitation program but rarely should be the sole intervention in the physical therapy office. Payers also recognize the benefits of active rehabilitation. As demonstrated in payment schedules, payers are more likely to reward the practice of exercise and hands-on manual therapy over the passive modalities.

Services to consider in addition to traditional physical therapy modalities and procedures include orthotics and work-injury rehabilitation and prevention programs. An orthotics service should be considered as an option when a relatively large orthopedic practice would serve as the referral base. A variety of custom and off-the-shelf products may be considered for inclusion in this program. A staff physical therapist, podiatrist, or a physician with a reputation and an expertise for treating the running population also contributes to the success of a foot orthotics program.

A work-injury rehabilitation and prevention program, including services such as work hardening, functional capacity evaluations, and preplacement screening, may make sense if a high volume of occupational health referrals is expected. A comprehensive work rehabilitation program will require a considerable amount of dedicated space to provide work-simulation services and employer-specific work equipment.

If, after a thorough situational analysis, the practice is poised to take advantage of the opportunities presented by an internal physical therapy department, it is important that the group remain aware of current state and national movements opposing physician-owned physical therapy services (POPTS). The American Physical Therapy Association (APTA) has a long-standing opposition to POPTS. It is engaged actively in developing and implementing strategies at the state and federal levels that would prohibit physician ownership of physical therapy services. The APTA is encouraging all its state chapters to establish a POPTS task force with a mission to prohibit POPTS. Delaware and South Carolina have interpreted statutes and enacted legislation that effectively prevents the employment of physical therapists by physicians. The concerns raised by the APTA and their state chapters include

1. Conflict of interest in which the patient's best interest may be compromised by the overuse of physical therapy services for the physician's financial gain

2. Loss of consumers' freedom of choice by limiting the patient's choice in choosing his or her own physical therapist
3. Financial harm to patients and third-party payors resulting from the economic impact of possible overuse

A frequently cited study supporting the APTA's position was published in the *Journal of the American Medical Association* in 1992. The study was conducted by the Florida Health Care Cost Containment Board in 1991 and examined "joint ventures" between health care professionals who made referrals and the entities that provided goods or services as a result of the referral. This study found higher utilization rates in joint ventures involving referrals to clinical laboratories, diagnostic imaging centers, and physical therapy clinics as compared with referrals to independents.

The American Association of Orthopaedic Surgeons has issued the following position statement in support of POPTS:

> The American Association of Orthopaedic Surgeons (AAOS) believes that patients should have access to quality, comprehensive and non-fragmented care. Doctors, nurses, physician's assistants, Physical Therapists and other health practitioners work together, often in the same office, to provide comprehensive care to patients. Separation of these services would only serve to disrupt a patient's treatment and further inconvenience them.
>
> The AAOS also believes that Physician Owned Physical Therapy Services should continue to be an alternative for patients. Patients should be given the ability to choose the site of care. Physicians employing Physical Therapists should communicate to the patient their financial interest in any physical therapy practice before referring the patient to the site. The physician should also discuss possible alternate sites for physical therapy services. In all instances, the AAOS believes that the best interest of the patient should be foremost when referring a patient for physical therapy services.

In conclusion, the successful internal physical therapy clinic will provide patients with accessible, high-quality, personal service. It will contribute positively to creating patient loyalty to and confidence in the physician and physical therapist.

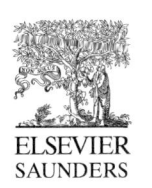

The Physician-Owned Occupational Health Department

Robert B. Weeks, BS, MT, MA

Minnesota Occupational Health, 1661 St. Anthony, St Paul, MN 55104, USA

The present author is the marketing director, customer service representative, and occupational health consultant for a profitable, physician-owned, freestanding occupational medicine program (OMP) owned by Summit Orthopedics, Ltd. Known as Minnesota Occupational Health (MOH), in St. Paul, Minnesota, the MOH program has existed since June 1997. MOH employs a staff of 22, including two board-certified occupational health physicians and three part-time emergency room physicians. In 6 years, the practice has grown from 0 patients on the first day to 120 per day; MOH became a profit center to Summit Orthopedics in less than 2 years. A key factor in this rapid growth is attributed to the author's previously established relationship with over 100 employers, as well as experience in marketing and sales for two major health systems in Minnesota. This article provides a process to evaluate the likelihood of establishing a financially viable OMP.

Preliminary assessments

Location

The location of a successful OMP must take into account market size, customer needs, accessibility, competitors, and availability of appropriate space. The decision of where to locate an OMP should not be made until marketing surveys have been completed. Until market potential is understood and competitors and their attributes have been identified, one should resist initial thoughts of integrating an OMP into an existing practice. Once this kind of analysis is complete, an informed decision can be made about the pros and cons of integration versus a free-standing occupational clinic site within the identified service area.

Quantifying the market potential

Most clients of an OMP will come from within a 15- to 20-minute drive time of the clinic. Establish a list of ZIP codes within this service area, then obtain the number of employers and employees within this area from the local library, through the Chamber of Commerce, or from the state's Department of Labor and Industry (or equivalent). MOH initially identified employer groups with more then 50 employees in order to focus its marketing efforts for the best return.

Posted on a state's Department of Labor Web site will be the frequency of injuries and illnesses per 100 full-time workers. Injury rates will vary by region and industry composition. Total recordable injury and illness cases have been declining nationwide since 1992 (decline of 23% between 1992 and 2001), and the number of injury and illnesses cases declined 9.8% from 2001 through 2002. Minnesota's workplace injury and illness rate stands at 5.3 cases per 100 full-time workers [1]. Workplace injuries have been reduced due to prevention activities, increased use of automation, and a decline in the number of manufacturing jobs. Employers have also been aggressive in managing their recordable injuries by working with providers to classify injuries as first-aid cases, which, according to guidelines established by the US Occupational Safety and Health Administration (OSHA), are nonrecordable.

Table 1 is an example of how to calculate an OMP's market potential. Use the state-specific rate of injuries and illnesses per 100 full-time workers. It is MOH's experience, as well as that

E-mail address: bweeks@summitortho.com

Table 1
Sample calculation for estimating injury visit

Factors to include in calculating market potential	Sample data
Total employers in area	16,061
Employers with > 50 employees	636
Number of employees of 636 employers	162,875 full-time employee (FTE)
Minnesota Department of Labor Statistics, 1996	7.8 injuries or illnesses per 100 FTE annually

Formula: Number of employees/100 FTE × number of illnesses × visits per injury = number of workers' compensation visits in market area
MOH 1996 numbers inserted 162,875/100 × 7.8 × 3.0 = 38,112 workers' compensation visits for MOH's market area annually adjusted for current injury rate data: 162,875/100 × 5.3 × 3 = 25,897 cases (32% reduction)

of others, that 2.5 to 3 visits per injury is the average (MOH's was 2.73 for 2002) [2].

At MOH, workers' compensation visits represent 44% of clinic visits but 54% of clinic revenue, with the balance of visits being physicals, drug testing, and immunizations. MOH currently averages 1800 visits per month. When calculating revenue per visit, one should refer to the allowable workers' compensation fees and the results of the competitor analysis for the pricing of employer-paid services such as physicals and drug testing.

Employer market survey

Once the names of the larger employers within the service area have been collected, the next step is the employer survey. It is critical to identify a mix of 100 employers, varying in size and industry, to obtain a statistically significant number on which to base assumptions. A minimum of 25% of the employers should be surveyed—both mail and telephone surveys can be used—but a phone survey is strongly recommended (remember, different employees at the companies may handle work injuries, physicals, and drug testing). Table 2 gives sample questions that can be asked as part of the employer survey. In the absence of a staff person familiar and comfortable with performing this type of survey, a marketing or advertising firm that specializes in health care marketing can be hired to perform this important data-gathering step. Such a firm can also help to develop survey questions and provide expertise in analyzing the results.

Once the market analysis and employer survey have been completed, a better understanding emerges of one's potential for success in the marketplace. There are also other customers who drive business, such as insurance companies, brokers, and managed care organizations, and these can also be surveyed.

Competitor survey

The employer survey should have identified which competitors employers are using for work injuries, physicals, and drug testing. Identifying a resource person in the insurance or broker industry is extremely helpful in gathering competitor information regarding services and pricing. Table 3 lists samples of questions for competitors.

Key service issues

The market survey data should provide a good understanding of the potential market and customer needs. Many of the items that appear in Table 2 were identified as essential services by and for employers and were built into MOH's program. Box 1 shows some key service issues not listed in the questionnaire but discovered during the phone interview (thus illustrating the benefits of this approach over a mailing a questionnaire).

Profit margins

In 1992 Ryan Associates, a nationally recognized occupational medicine educational provider, and Occupational Health Research, a nationally recognized occupational health research group, conducted a national study of the types of OMPs (Table 4). One hundred nineteen occupational programs were studied, and the profit margins found in this study varied from 4.6% to 9.8% [2]. On the basis of MOH's experience (ie, with appropriate staffing and motivated medical staff), the margins found in this study are extremely low. In the same study, the three top revenue generators in an occupational health setting are injury treatment, preplacement examinations, and drug testing, followed in

Table 2
Employer market survey sample questions

How many FTE employees do you have?
How many shifts do you operate?
Do you have a number of employees that use public transportation?
Number of recordable work related injuries for the previous year.
If an employee has a work-related injury, where would you send him/her?
Do you receive same-day communication back from the provider? Is this important for you?
Would having an in-clinic orthopedic specialist to facilitate specialty care when needed be important to you?
Do you perform replacement physicals? (If no, skip next question)
Can you schedule physicals within 24 hours? Is this important to you?
Do you perform drug testing and under what circumstances (federal and or non-federal)
Are you required to have DOT examinations?
Is easy access to free parking for trucks important to you? Length of trucks?
Do you do preplacement and/or annual audiograms (at the clinic or at company site)?
Do you do positions that require the use of respirators?
If a new occupational health provider were available in your service area, under what circumstances would you consider changing providers?

Table 3
Competitor analysis

Type of service	Service cost	Notes
Breath alcohol test		
Pulmonary function test		
Respiratory examination		
DOT initial examination		
DOT drug test		
Non-DOT drug test—5 panel		
Non-DOT drug test—7 panel		
Hepatitis B vaccination		
History and physical		
Audiogram		
Preplacement examination		
Urine drug collection only		

Service requirements	Notes
Response time to set up meeting	
Physicals scheduled up until—(time)	
After-hour care offered?	
Number of clinic sites	
Number of board-certified occupational medicine physicians	
Task-specific preplacement exams	
Walk-in injury care available	
Specialist referrals tracked how	
Pharmacy services direct billing	
Injury care dictated notes sent	
On-site company visits	
What on-site manager/employee training programs offered	
Preplacement scheduling (24–72 h)	
Convenient location/easy to locate	
Free parking	

descending order by rehabilitation, workplace consulting, on-site nursing, wellness, and employee assistance programs [2].

Planning the clinic operation

Location

Location and staffing are important. MOH has easy access off the freeway—between Minneapolis and St. Paul—and occupies about half the second floor, encompassing around 3000 ft^2. MOH sees 90 to 150 patients per day, with two medical providers, four front-desk staff, six medical assistants, one medical records assistant, a staff of four for on-site and after-hour services, one marketing person, one claims management person and two administrative assistants. MOH has seven examination rooms for injury care and physicals; one treatment room for lacerations; one x-ray room; and four rooms for workup of physicals, where vision, audiometric, and respirator testing are performed. In addition, there are two specially designed bathrooms for the collection of drug tests to comply with federal drug collection requirements.

The MOH building houses support services for Summit Orthopedics' six clinics and three surgical center. Support services include centralized scheduling, physical therapy, an MRI scanner, management information systems staff, and billing. These services were relocated from rented locations to MOH at a much lower cost per square foot. In addition to lower cost, the entire network of orthopedic clinics can easily access support services; parking is free.

> **Box 1. Additional key service issues as identified during phone interviews**
>
> - Providing immediate access for new injuries (when reported by worker to employer)
> - Coordinating after-hour care where the clinic has access to medical records
> - Writing appropriate restrictions and letting the employers find work within those restrictions (avoiding lost time)
> - Providing access to interpreters for non–English-speaking patients
> - Making medical forms available in Spanish
> - Locating clinic on a bus route
> - Notifying employers of patient no-shows
> - Having physicians call on lost-time injuries
> - Providing on-site or coordinated services for rehabilitation
> - Providing notification of physical results on same day of examination
> - Making bills that are clear and easy to read
> - Having physicians who are willing to go on company site visits

When considering space in an existing clinic, take into account potential market growth and the company's needs (as identified in the market survey). If the OMP is to be integrated into an existing practice, because of the specialized requirements and knowledge of an occupational medicine practice, the reception area should be staffed separately, with a well-defined intake and discharge area for the occupational health customers.

Equipment needs

On the basis of the customer needs survey, the clinic will have identified clients that require special service needs and specialized equipment. Such equipment includes spirometry for respirator clearance, x-ray equipment for taking standardized B reader films for asbestos exposure, a retrofitted bathroom with an outside shutoff with no sink (as required for federal drug collections), breath alcohol-testing machine for US Department of Transportation (DOT) testing, and audiometric testing when companies come under OSHA-hearing conservation requirements. All of the specialized equipment or testing mentioned here requires specific training and certification of staff performing the testing (Table 5).

Management information systems support and billing

When integrating a practice, it would not be uncommon to consider integrating its existing billing system for the use of the occupational medicine services. However, this has proven to be futile and, in one larger hospital system, extremely

Table 4
Make up of occupational medicine programs 1992

Hospital/emergency department based	30 (25.2%)
Hospital/nonemergency based	29 (24.4%)
Hospital/freestanding	34 (28.6%)
Non-hospital/freestanding	13 (10.9%)
Other	13 (10.9%)

From Workplace injuries and illnesses for 2002. U.S. Department of Labor, Bureau of Labor Statistics. Available at: http://www.bls.gov/news.release/pdf/osh.pdf. Accessed February 23, 2004.

Table 5
Estimated specialized equipment costs

Special equipment needed	Number to order	Cost per item ($)
Breath alcohol testing (DOT approved)[a]	2	2800–4000 each
Microprocessor for audiometric testing[a]	1	3800–6500
Audio sound booth	1	3800–8000
Spirometer[a]	1	2300–3200
Vision tester with color plates	2	1800–2300 each
Power exam table with arm board for lacerations	1	7500–10,500
Yearly license fee for specialized Systoc software		19,000–21,000

[a] Specialized training and certification for medical assistants' use of this equipment are required but may not be readily available. Costs will vary depending on location of training and travel costs. Some of the certification programs last for 2 days. Estimated cost of training, excluding travel, is $2000 per employee.

expensive; instead, the hospital opted for software designed for occupational medicine functions. SYSTOC [3] (Occupational Health Resources, Skowhegan, ME) is an example of specialized occupational health system software. The system integrates billing and scheduling, functions as an order-entry system specific to company needs, and provides task-specific worksheets for nursing, with reporting criteria. SYSTOC also has an injury-tracking component, which can be used in case management.

In its market environment, MOH has added new clients a number of times because competitors have tried to use existing systems within their practices, with the result that they produced illegible and inaccurate bills to companies—a source of much dissatisfaction to employers. With specialty computer software such as SYSTOC available at a reasonable cost, it makes little sense to invest the time and effort into "tinkering" with non-occupational software. Also, the ongoing updates and changes required within the occupational health environment are available from a dedicated occupational health software provider.

Staffing

When MOH opened its doors in June 1997, it employed one occupational health physician, a backup emergency department (ER) physician, two receptionists, three medical assistants, two marketing staff (one of whom was half time), one billing specialist, and a transcriptionist. All of the employees had worked in occupational medicine clinics for a number of years and brought valuable knowledge to the practice.

Spending the time to identify and recruit staff with knowledge and excellent customer service skills is critical to a successful OMP. Early in the planning stages, key people to be recruited must be identified based on the employer surveys.

According to the market survey conducted by Ryan Associates and Occupational Health Resources, "the lack of medical staff support was rated as the most important barrier in establishing a successful program," followed by lack of effective billing procedures, insufficient staff, well-entrenched competition, lack of administrative support, and insufficient space/parking [2]. Recruiting an occupational medicine physician can add credibility to a program, especially from an employer's perspective, because of the valuable knowledge such a physician has in the areas of workers' compensation and OSHA regulations.

The right occupational medicine physician must also have the customer service skills and desire to accommodate the needs of all customers, including employers, insurers, case managers, and patients. He or she must have excellent communication skills, be flexible, be able to write appropriate return-to-work restrictions, and be equally available to the patient and other customers. Besides consulting with employers on workplace health and safety concerns, the occupational medicine physician must be a hard-working clinician with the ability to see a substantial patient caseload—up to 45 patients a day. This single issue is a marginal one, or one in which profits can exceed 15%.

An excellent supplement for the occupational medicine physician is a board-certified ER physician. Having an ER physician available raises the level of expertise available for walk-in patients with acute injuries. An additional benefit gained by using ER physicians from a local hospital is the follow-up visits that can be captured from injuries that occur on second and third shifts. The local employer groups also benefit from the ER physician by working with the occupational medicine physician at the clinic (eg, writing appropriate return-to-work orders). Building a successful OMP involves nurturing and integrating relationships that benefit the injured worker and the employer.

When recruiting medical assistants for occupational health services, specialized training is required (see Table 5). Finding qualified staff is not easy, but it is a worthwhile effort because having experienced staff familiar with the testing procedures lends credibility to a newly established program.

Marketing the occupational medicine program

Strength, weakness, opportunity, and threat analysis

After gathering all of the information obtained in the market research, a strength, weakness, opportunity, and threat (SWOT) analysis of the program should be performed. Table 6 lists some of the items that MOH identified within its program.

Marketing and sales overview

The marketing strategy should focus on the clinic's strengths and implemented opportunities. For instance, MOH offers an integrated delivery service, or in simple terms, "one-stop shopping," to its customers (employers, employees, third-party administrators insurers, and brokers).

Table 6
Strength, weakness, opportunity, and threat analysis: strengths

Strengths	Specifics
Central location and access	Easy access from major freeways
	Free parking
	Open lot with space for small/large trucks
Strong, successful sales staff	Knowledgeable business health consultants with diverse knowledge of buyer's regulatory compliance issues (eg, DOT, substance abuse testing, OSHA regulations)
Link with orthopedic specialists	Available in-clinic orthopedic specialists
	Coordination of medical records and return-to-work among in-house orthopedic specialists
	On-site rehabilitation (physical therapist)
	In-clinic MRI equipment
Customer-focused attitude	Timely, thorough communication, both written and verbal
	Customized programs and services
	Responsive to customer needs
SWOT analysis: weaknesses	
Single-site location	Less attractive to multiple-site employers
After-hours systems access	Lack of integrated after-hours injury care
SWOT analysis: opportunities	
MIS capabilities (Systoc)	Central patient database
	Client dial-in capabilities
	Electronic billing
	Enhanced management reporting
Referrals from occupational health for ancillary services	Physical therapy
	Orthopedic consults' and surgery
	MRI scans
Jointly sponsored education seminars for employers	Summit orthopedic joint musculoskeletal education
	Joint newsletters
SWOT analysis: threats	
Legislative changes	Reduction in workers' compensation fee schedule
	Reduction in disability compensation
Single-payer systems	
Competing area occupational health programs	

All customers benefit by receiving timely communication, responsive treatment, and a consolidated bill and medical record for all needed services. These services include initial treatment assessment, triage and referral to in-house orthopedic specialist when needed, rehabilitation, radiology, laboratory, surgical, and employer-paid services.

With respect to sales, tools and promotional materials need to be developed, such as a brand name and logo, a brochure with a logo, fact sheets outlining the services offered, and well-laid-out maps with clear directions to the clinic (also directions to the clinic via public transportation, such as bus routes). It is unnecessary to spend a significant amount of money developing sales materials or a logo. MOH's budget for this activity was less than $10,000, which included printing of all collateral support material (eg, letterhead, business cards, maps, phone directory, and service fact sheets). Knowledgeable sales professionals will complete the sale, and the printed materials will mainly be used to summarize key points of service. It is the author's experience that most-used collateral support material will be the following:

- A clear map on how to get to the clinic, including address, hours, bus route, and phone number for appointments
- Laminated wall map with tear-off sheets for injury care, with the same information as above
- Staff directory with phone numbers for all services
- A Web site (a recent addition at MOH)

A word of caution regarding using mass mailings as a marketing tool: use this approach sparingly, if at all, because of the limited response that typically is received, the cost, and the inability to follow up in a timely manner. Prospective clients are just too occupied today and, like many people, tend to discard such mailings into "the round file." The best approach is highly likely to be targeted sales, as suggested by the market research. Another simple (yet effective) marketing approach is to drive around the service area—a process the author calls "prospecting"—identifying potential customers, making phone contacts, and following up with a written proposal.

Advertising

Target advertising to resources that are read and used by target customers. The following are sources of advertising that MOH has found to be effective: display ads in the Yellow Pages, listed under "occupational medicine," covering the service area, and display ads in locally distributed trade journals and the Chamber of Commerce's yearly publication.

A Web site can serve as a portal for targeted customers by providing information helpful to their business.

Financial considerations

As a new start-up OMP, MOH had an initial outlay of around $100,000 for equipment and supplies, excluding the cost of space. Its business plan called for a break-even point in around 2.5 years; it was achieved by the end of the second year. Besides the initial outlay for equipment, and taking into account the cost of space, MOH experienced a negative cash flow of around $300,000 before revenues equaled costs, beginning in the 14th month of operations. By the beginning of the third year, MOH had broken even and paid back the initial investment.

According to Dr. William Newkirk, every dollar generated in a free-standing facility for injury care treatment will generate $3.50 for outpatient services, $1.40 for inpatient services, and $1.60 for physician referral services [4]. MOH's experience in the year ending 2002 was that it captured $0.62 as spin-off revenue for every dollar of workers' compensation revenue. This spin-off revenue was to the following departments: physical therapy ($0.24), MRI ($0.11), X ray ($0.8), and $0.19 for orthopedic referrals. The profit margins addressed earlier by the author do not take into account any spin-off revenues. It is not practical to be able to capture all revenue opportunities. Each additional service has to be evaluated based on customer needs and the ability to provide that service cost effectively (eg, after-hour injuries care). Summit Orthopedics is in the process of evaluating whether to replace its current MRI scanner with one capable of scanning backs. This is an example of a benefit derived from being part of a large orthopedic practice, as MOH could not justify solely owning an MRI scanner.

Opportunities in occupational medicine in the current environment

Background

Musculoskeletal disorders—an employer and endemic public health burden

Musculoskeletal disorders (MSDs) involving strains and sprains represent the leading nature of injuries and illnesses in American industry. Of cases of days away from work as a result of strains and sprains, 31% involve employees with less than 1 year of on-the-job experience [4].

For the year 2000, there were 578,000 MSDs. The preceding six years, sprains and strains represented nearly half the nonfatal occupational injuries and illnesses (31% from overexertion) involving days away from work. Principally, the back was the most affected by disabling work incidents in almost every industry division. However, upper and lower extremity strains and sprains were significantly involved as well [5].

Liberty Mutual Insurance Company's 1998 internal claims database reconfirms these data. A study of its own losses showed that overexertion injuries and illnesses topped the list of the 10 leading causes of workplace claims, at a cost of about $9 billion to all employers nationwide [6].

The number of lost work-time injuries and illnesses has been steadily decreasing since 1992; the percentage of MSDs to total incidents does not appear to have been affected. MSDs have become a serious public health burden by affecting the ability of American enterprise to safely staff the multitude of physically demanding jobs, with no apparent end in sight.

Experience modification ratings

There is increasing pressure on employers to reduce their workers' compensation costs owing to work-related injuries in order to reduce their experience modification ratings. This, in turn, reduces the cost for workers' compensation insurance. Where employers are self-insured, any reduction in savings on medical costs from work-related injuries goes directly to their bottom line. This also reduces their experience modification rating.

The experience modification rating involves a complex formula devised by workers' compensation insurers, which takes into account the incidence and frequency of injuries that occur in the workplace. The resultant rating is calculated over a period of 3 years, so changes that companies make in reducing costs related to work injuries will not show up in a reduced rating for several years. Similar types of employers are then compared with one another and are used as a comparison to determine how well they manage these costs as a result of work injuries. A company that has an experience modification rating of 1.0 would have costs similar to others in the industry. If a company has a rating of 1.2, its costs are 20% higher than a company with a 1.0 rating in the same industry. On the other hand, a company with a rating of 0.08 would have costs 20% below the average.

The importance of this is twofold. The more obvious is where a company has an experience modification rating of less then 1.0. As a result, it has less overhead because of decreased insurance costs, allowing the company to be more competitive in its bidding process. This reduction in incidences not only shows up in reduced insurance costs, but also in increased productivity owing to fewer work stoppages as a result of work injuries. The second issue relates to the way corporations—requesting bids for construction projects—look at bidders. Corporations are looking for contractors with competitive bids, but, just as important, they are looking for contractors that will complete projects on time and in a safe manner. Corporations, or contractors, do not want to be in the morning headlines announcing an accident that may involve a death as a result of work injury. Such an incident results in a project being shut down and an immediate investigation by OSHA, which is time consuming and costly for all involved.

Employers are aggressively managing their OSHA-recordable injuries to be competitive within the marketplace. An OSHA-recordable injury results when an injured worker is not capable of returning to work and performing the full essential functions of the job as he or she did before the work-related injury. OSHA-recordable injuries can also depend on the type of medical treatment ordered by the treating physician, regardless of whether the injured worker returns to work and performs full functions. An example of an OSHA-recordable injury in this situation would be when the physician orders physical therapy or prescribes a prescription medication—either one of these modalities or treatments automatically results in an injury becoming recordable.

The need for employers to reduce their experience modification rating and OSHA-recordable injuries is becoming a business necessity to obtain contracts. Builders of commercial developments not only look at the contractor's bid for the work, they also take a hard look at a company's experience modification rating and its OSHA-recordable injuries. Contractors have lost bids for projects—even when their fees are lower—to another bidder whose fees are higher but with a lower experience modification rating and/or fewer OSHA-recordable injuries. Owners of companies are holding their safety people responsible for preventing injuries and aggressively managing their return-to-work and OSHA-recordable injuries. The compensation and continued employment of safety personnel depend on their success in managing injury claims and OSHA- recordable injuries.

The occupational medicine quandaries and opportunities

The first quandary is that a physician who treats work-related injuries has not only the patient as a customer, but also the employer. The physician needs to reduce OSHA-recordable injuries while providing appropriate medical care. The employer wants a fully productive employee, but the worker might require returning to restricted-duty work until he or she is ready for full-duty work.

This scenario can result in conflicts with the treating physician and the employer. Over the years, physicians have been trained to practice as the patient's advocate, often not hearing the pleas of employers for help in managing OSHA-recordable claims. To be successful today in occupational medicine, a physician must wear these "two hats" without compromising patient care. The physician must have an open line of communication with the employer regarding return-to-work issues and treatment plans, and patients must be managed in a timely manner if the physician is to maintain a successful practice.

A second quandary occurs in a combined practice, where there is an occupational medicine department and independent specialty physicians, such as orthopedics, who see patients for work-related injuries from other primary care systems. Often in this situation, the specialist ignores the requests of employers or does not communicate with the employer. The physician who relies on information solely from the patient falls into the trap of being a patient advocate only. The employer's concerns regarding return-to-work orders are ignored, resulting in OSHA-recordable injuries. In a combined practice such as this, even though a specialist physician is in a separate department, he or she is "guilty by association."

Attention to this issue is especially crucial in states where the patient has freedom of choice in providers. In one example, the occupational medicine department agrees to see not only work-related injuries for a company, but it also performs physical examinations or other mandated examinations under DOT or OSHA, which generate revenues in excess of $25,000 per year. An injured employee from this company goes to another primary care provider, outside the combined occupational medicine practice, but is referred to one of the specialty orthopedic physicians, who ignores the employer's concerns of early return-to-work or the management of OSHA-related claims. As a result of this scenario, the employer becomes disenchanted with the occupational medicine department. Although the occupational medicine department has no control over this situation, the employer believes it should have, as the department is part of a single organization. As a result, the employer moves its business to another occupational medicine provider. In this example, the occupational medicine department has "won the battle, but lost the war."

Summary comments

In a perfect world, all injured workers are highly motivated to get back to work as soon as medically feasible and are willing to ignore the minor aches and pains that happened with any injury. The injured workers are dedicated to their employer and want it to succeed in becoming an employer advocate when being treated for a work injury. Non–work-related incidents are never confused with a personal injury outside the workplace. An injured worker reminds the treating physician that prescribing a medication will result in their employer incurring an OSHA-recordable injury, and ask whether an over-the-counter medication, such as ibuprofen, may work just as well.

Of course, it is not a perfect world. And sometimes, in around 3% to 5% of cases, the injured worker has other motives—sometimes not intentionally but as a fault of the system or circumstances. The following hypothetical example will help to clarify this point. A worker is performing demanding work at minimum wage or slightly above. He also works for an employer who is very demanding and hardly ever praises employees for the things they do right, yet is quick to point out their faults. This employee has obligations at home, such as children; his significant other works at a minimum wage job, and together they have daycare expenses. The employee may also carry disability insurance, which may cover certain expenses if he is disabled because of a work-related injury.

The system for compensation of work-related injuries allows for this injured employee to receive 66% of his income—tax free—if he is unable to work because of a work-related injury. This will vary from state to state, but the author is using Minnesota as an example. In this situation, the injured worker may be at home taking over care of the children, avoiding daycare expenses, while having other obligations taken care of by disability insurance. Financially, he is further ahead than if gainfully employed. The system, depending on the state, allows a worker to report an injury that, although it may have happened in the past, is still covered when reported in the future. This injury may have occurred at work or at home, but is still allowed to be claimed as work related.

With the ever-increasing age of today's workforce, older workers just cannot perform the demands of a physically taxing job as they did when they were younger. As a result, there is a tendency for more work-related injuries. The obesity rate in the United States also is rising, and being out of shape is a contributing factor in work-related or non–work-related injuries.

The abuse of illegal or legal drugs is of concern for 5% to 10% of the population. Various addictive types of drugs are more available, such as methamphetamine or marijuana—a newer form of which is referred to as "British Columbia Grown" and is many times more potent than what was available in the 1960s. There is a current trend among teenagers in having what they call "pharming parties," where they take accessible prescribed medications from their parents, bring them to parties, and exchange and take them knowing little of the consequences.

The solution to these situations is beyond the scope of this article, but is something that as a society needs to be addressed. Any of these or their combination contributes to work-related injuries.

Opportunities

As the result of the circumstances mentioned above, a progressive **OMP** can partner with employers to help diminish the impact of these situations that contribute to work-related injuries.

Preplacement physicals

There are various levels of physical examinations available to the physician, as a tool to identify medical conditions, that may impact the applicant's ability to perform the essential function of the job. Physical examinations can be a tool in reducing injuries, provided that jobs for which applicants are applying require a significant amount of physical demands.

As a starting point, the occupational medicine clinic should review the lost-run reports from the employer's workers' compensation carrier. These reports describe in detail the types and frequency of injuries that the employer has incurred. Preplacement examinations will not prevent injuries that result from poor safety practices. Physical examinations can, however, identify pre-existing conditions that may impact the person's ability to perform the essential functions of the job. Once the loss-run reports have been analyzed, and it is determined that some injuries were due to pre-existing conditions, a preplacement examination can help to identify appropriate candidates for the job. The level or degree of the examination depends on the work demands.

Traditionally—and in most common practice today—the physical is where the applicant completes a medical history questionnaire that includes a detailed history of past medical problems, treatments, surgeries, and compensation from previous work injuries or disability claims. This examination will also check a person's vitals, including height, weight, blood pressure, vision, and a urine analysis to detect the presence of glucose, which may indicate undiagnosed diabetes. The physical also includes a complete head-to-toe examination by the physician, who looks for abnormalities, scars, hernias, and other medical conditions that may affect the person's ability to perform the job. The examining physician depends on the applicant providing an accurate history of past problems. Unfortunately, this is not always the case, and the applicant will not disclose some pre-existing conditions, which may in fact disqualify him or her from obtaining the job. (It has been MOH's experience that an applicant can hide pre-existing conditions if the goal is to obtain a job.) The physical is a valuable tool, though, for identifying conditions, such as uncontrolled high blood pressure, possible diabetes, or the presence of a hernia. The flexibility evaluation or the presence of unexplained scars may tip off the physician to ask additional questions to flush out past medical conditions.

The basic physical examination, as described above, is a good starting place. However, as pointed out, there are limitations, especially if the applicant withholds information regarding previous medical conditions. In addition, the applicant is seen for a brief period of time, and it is difficult to assess the person's ability to perform demanding tasks over an extended period of time. It behooves the employer, where work tasks are physically demanding, to not overlook the next level of evaluating applicants, which involves work simulation or strength testing.

Work simulation/lifting-capacity testing

There are two types of lifting-capacity testing that have been used as a measurement of an individual's capacity to perform the physical demands for essential job requirements:

A. The Isernhagen method for determining functional capacity involves having job applicants perform a series of tasks, under the observation of a trained occupational or physical therapist, which simulate the essential functions of the job. This often is done in a warehouse situation and requires about an hour of an applicant's time. This process and its validation have recently been discussed in the journal *Spine* [7].

B. The Isokinetic methodology for functional capacity determination involves the use of a dynamometer, where the strength of the individual's arms, legs, and back is evaluated. These strength determinations are then rated against the strength required by the job for various essential job tasks. This testing requires about 20 minutes of the applicant's time and can be performed in a clinic. The Code of Federal Regulations [8] addresses strength and agility testing and the rights of employers to use such testing for pre-employment evaluation. It is absolutely acceptable to require a candidate to demonstrate that he or she is able to perform the required essential functions of the job.

Pre-employment strength and agility testing is permitted under the Americans with Disabilities Act, as long as it is not discriminatory. After a job offer has been made, employers may perform medical and nonmedical strength and agility testing and inquire as to disabilities. If the testing becomes discriminatory in nature when denying candidates on the basis of test results, the employer must show that the tasks of business necessity are directly related to the job. The most protective manner to show business necessity is to have jobs evaluated by a third-party professional ergonomist for strength and agility task requirements.

In the case of injury during the physical agility testing, one must look to the case law of that particular state, because some states will grant workers' compensation benefits and some will not.

MOH uses both forms of functional capacity testing. There is a trend with employers preferring the Isokinectic approach, as it requires not only less time, but also can be easily accommodated at one location. Isokinectic testing also allows the clinic to have results immediately after the testing, so that a qualified candidate can be available to work on completion of the evaluation. The timeliness of the agility results is a crucial factor in helping employers to place an applicant in a job as soon as feasible. A typical scenario at MOH is same-day access, whereby candidates who meet the criteria are available to work that same day.

Drug testing

Background

The following discussion is based on a breakdown of positive drug results shown in Table 7.

In 2002, Medtox Laboratories tested 1,637,257 specimens for the presence of illegal or controlled substances, and of these, 91,538 were positive (5.59% positive rate).

The effects of drug use, the increased incidence in the use of health care benefits, increased absenteeism, and involuntary turnover rate (47%) were well documented in a study performed by the US Postal Service [9].

Many employers have implemented drug testing for preplacement screening, reasonable suspicion testing, postaccident testing, and random testing for safety-sensitive positions to reduce the incidence of work-related injuries and absenteeism as well as to increase productivity. As more employers use this tool to develop a safe work environment, those who do not draw from a pool of people where the incidence of drug use is less prevalent may incur more risks.

Employers implementing drug testing should have a clear written policy about testing. In addition, employers have to be sure that their testing complies with any state statutes. Any employer embarking on drug testing is strongly advised to consult with a legal representative first.

Discussion

The occupational medicine clinic is in an excellent position to work with its clients to ensure that the testing program implemented is effective and efficient. There is a large variety of drug panels from which to choose when implementing drug testing. Box 2 provides recommendations

Table 7
Testing for US Department of Transportation (5 versus other panels)

Drug	Total number	Total positive (%)	Total tests (%)
THC positives	51,092	55.8	3.10
Cocaine positives	17,358	19.0	1.10
Amphetamine positives	6868	7.5	0.41
Opiate positives	5811	6.3	0.35
PCP positives	1025	1.1	0.06
Barbiturate positives	1833	2.0	0.11
Benzodiazepine positives	2995	3.3	0.18
Propoxyphene positives	3444	3.8	0.21
Methadone positives	757	0.8	0.05
Methaqualone positives	355	0.4	0.02

5 DOT drugs = 5.02% positive rate (89.8% of all positives)
5 Non-DOT drugs = 0.57% positive rate
1,637,257 specimens tested in the year 2002
91,538 total positives (5.59% positive rate)
Does not include alcohol positives

Abbreviations: PCP, phencyclidine; THC, marijuana.
Data from Medtox Laboratories, Jim Pederson, 402 West County Road D, St. Paul, MN 55112, Phone: 1-800-832-3244, 651-636-7466.

Box 2. Minnesota Occupational Health recommendations for implementation of a drug testing program

1. Employers should identify clinics that employ certified collectors—as required by the DOT—and perform drug collections, as a core part of their business. This is extremely important, as any documentation errors occurring during the collection may invalidate the testing process.
2. The occupational medicine clinic should also obtain a copy of the company's policy to ensure that the testing being performed complies with the company policy. MOH has found that employer's policies do not fully address the presence of adulterants in urine or diluted samples (often as a result of an attempt by the donor to adulterate or hide the presence of drugs). Several products are commercially available that may be used to attempt to mask the presence of drugs.
3. All samples being screened for the presence of drugs should include a testing panel for the presence of adulterant, either at the time of collection or when the testing is performed by the laboratory. All laboratories offer this option, but the employer or the occupational medicine clinic working with that employer has to request this battery of tests. MOH uses a commercially available testing strip to test for the presence of adulterants and diluted specimens. If an adulterant is found, these samples are referred to the certified laboratory for confirmation. Medtox was among the first to publish findings regarding extremely diluted specimens [10]. Medtox found in this study that urine specimens submitted for employment drug testing were extremely diluted compared with those submitted to their laboratory for other types of testing. Medtox also found that a high proportion of excessively diluted specimens contained controlled substances below the screening detection levels used by laboratories.
4. For reasonable suspicion testing, a company should use an expanded drug-testing panel, which includes illegal drugs and prescription drugs that can be used illegally (use of a drug without a prescription). All employers incorporating reasonable suspicion as a part of their testing should have their supervisors attend a training class that provides them with the appropriate methods in identifying possible drug users, including the process for appropriate documentation to avoid any legal issues. These classes typically last from 2 to 3 hours.
5. A company should consider using a DOT-certified medical review officer (MRO) for all drug testing. All DOT testing requires the use of an MRO, whereas many states do not require this for non-DOT testing. (MOH uses a DOT-certified MRO for all drug testing.) The role of the MRO is to contact the donor—before the results of the drug test are released to the employer—to validate any prescription drug the donor may be taking, as legally prescribed. As a result, the MRO may turn a positive test into a negative report.
6. The applicant should be offered a position where drug testing is mandatory and be required to have the drug test done within 24 to 48 hours of the offer. The reason for this time period is that many drugs clear the system within a short period of time (Table 8).
7. The company's alcohol-testing policy should address what constitutes a positive test. Many states have legal limits for driving, but employers may elect to have a zero-tolerance policy in the workplace and, as a result, have lower limits than those legally required to drive a motor vehicle.
8. A company should consider establishing a relationship with a substance abuse professional. (MOH helps its clients with such a relationship.) The substance abuse professional evaluates a current employee, recommends appropriate treatment, and coordinates a return to work. Employees' rights vary from state to state, but in some states, for a first positive drug test the employee has to be given the right to rehabilitation before he or she can be terminated. Through experience MOH has learned how important

this is to have in place and to thus avoid the call from the employer asking, "I have a positive drug test, what do I do?"

9. A company should have access to drug test results after normal business hours. MOH provides an on-site collection service 24 hours a day, any day of the week, to help its clients to conform to their drug-testing requirements outside of normal business hours. Many employers will also use this service as a convenience for reasonable suspicion testing, as this obviates the need to have a supervisor transport a donor to the clinic. This can be arranged ahead of time (eg, when an employer knows this situation will be addressed with an employee). This service is a valuable tool in a most difficult situation.

that MOH suggests for employers when implementing their drug testing program.

Customer retention

Retention requires a coordinated team effort to produce outcomes that meet customer expectations. The present author has never seen a satisfied customer go elsewhere for service. As easy as this may sound, it becomes a challenge for management to instill the importance of customer satisfaction and striving to meet customer needs 100% of the time. This is vital for continued growth. In an occupational medicine setting, a single dissatisfied customer may result in tens of thousands of dollars in lost revenue. In a primary care setting, a dissatisfied patient means losing a single patient; in occupational medicine, having a dissatisfied employer could mean losing hundreds of patients. Clearly written, well-understood, and measurable compliance to policies and procedures is critical to consistent quality service. Good policy compliance will minimize variation and produce a more consistent outcome.

Staff orientation to customer needs, as identified from the employer survey, becomes an important training tool for employee orientation. In addition, a mechanism should be in place to measure desired outcomes. A good example of a customer requirement is the ability to schedule physicals within 24 hours so as to have the applicant evaluated and available for work as soon as feasible. Correspondingly, a measurable clinic outcome is to report physical results back to the employer on the day of the examination. In an integrated team approach, it is not just one person's responsibility to make sure physicals are reported but that of the whole care team. Every person, every day is responsible for the continuous success of the OMP.

Much has been written regarding continuous quality improvement (CQI) and total quality management, both of which assume that quality is determined by meeting or exceeding customer needs. It continues to be elusive just what specific training, background, upbringing, or education instills in an individual the drive to meet customer needs. It occurs from the satisfaction of a job well done or from a simple "thank you" from a customer whose needs have just been met. Ryder and Newkirk [11] sum this up nicely:

> However, the fact is that CQI is not a program at all; rather, it is a way of thinking, a way of being, a way of doing business. CQI involves no magic; many successful clinics already use CQI tools and philosophies without the label and fanfare that currently accompany CQI program implementation.

Summary

This article has discussed opportunities in which the occupational medicine clinic can partner with employers to help them to reduce the occurrence of work-related injuries and provide a safer work environment. This article does not attempt to cover all issues—employers must address safety and ergonomic issues within the workplace as well. The occupational health clinic should be a readily available resource for any of these issues.

In the practice of occupational medicine, the traditional role of the medical practitioner, in which the patient is the primary focus, is expanded. A successful OMP involves developing a partnership with employers, insurers, brokers, third-party administrators, qualified rehabilitation counselors, case managers, specialty referral physicians, pharmacies, and hospital systems beyond patient care. With smaller employer groups, occupational health is often used for management of workplace health and safety needs, including ergonomics and prevention services.

Table 8
Controlled substances—uses and effects

Drugs	Trade or other names	Detection period
Opiates		
Opium	Dover's powder, paregoric, laudanum	1–2 d
Morphine	Morphine, roxanol, roxanol-SR	1–2 d
Codeine	Tylenol with codeine, Empirin with codeine, Robitussen A-C, Florinal with codeine	1–2 d
Heroin	Diacetylmorphine, horse, smack, dragon's tail	1–2 d
Hydromorphone	Dilaudid	1–2 d
Meperidine	Demerol, mepergan, pethidine	1–2 d
Methadone	Dolophine, methadone	5–10 d
Oxycodone	Percodan, Percocet, Tylox	8–24 h
Other opiates	Numorphan, Tussionex, Fenanyl, Darvon, Lomotil, Talwin	8–24 h
Depressants		
Alcohol	Beer, wine, liquor	6–10 h
Barbiturates	Amytal, Butisol, Fiorinal, Membutal, Seconal, Tuinal, Phenobarbital, black beauties	2–10 d
Benzodiazepines	Ativan, Dalmane, Diazepam, Librium, Xanax, Serax, Valium, Tranxene, Versed, Halcion, Paxipam, Restoril	1–6 wk
Methaqualone	Quaalude	2 wk
Glutethimide	Doriden	2–10 d
Other Depressants	Equanil, Miltown, Noludar, Placidyl, soma, chloral hydrate	2–7 d
Stimulants		
Cocaine	Coke, flake, snow, crack	2–4 d
Amphetamines	Biphematine, Delcobase, Desoxyn, Dexedrine, Obetrol, reds	1–2 d
Phenmetrazine	Preludin	1–2 d
Methylphenidate	Ritalin	1–2 d
Nicotine	Cigarettes, chewing, tobacco, cigars	2–4 d
Other Stimulants	Adipex, Cylert, Didrex, Ionamin, Plegine, Tenuate, Tepanil, Prelu-2	1–2 d
Hallucinogens		
LSD (lysergic acid diethylamide	Acid, microdot	8 h
Mescaline	Mesc, buttons, cactus, peyote	2–3 d
Amphetamine variants	2,5—DMA; PMA; STP; MDA; MDMA; TMA; DOM; DOB	8–24 h
Phencyclidine	PCP, angel dust, hog	2–8 d
Marijuana	Pot, Acapulco gold, grass, reefer, sinsemilla, Thai sticks	2 d–11 wk
Tetrahydrocannabinol	THC, Marinol	2 d–11 wk
Hashish, hashish oil	Hash	2 d–11 wk
Other hallucinogens	Bufotenine, Ibogaine, DMT, DET, psilocybin, psilocin, PCE, PCPy, TCP	6 h

A successful OMP must continue to monitor the changing needs of its customers through periodic meetings and surveys. As new technologies are developed and laws change, employers must be educated. In this age of cost containment and escalating health care costs, occupational programs have to evolve into proactive programs that assist employers with more of their workplace employment needs as they pertain to prevention, cost containment, physicals, drug testing, and mandated compliance examinations.

With nationwide declining injury rates, OMPs must look to new sources of employer-paid services. A recently added service at MOH is the provision of drug testing needs on a nationwide basis. Each market is unique, a product of the employer mix, nature of competition, and changes in workers' compensation laws. Therefore, there is no one model program that is an exact fit for any particular market.

References

[1] U.S. Department of Labor. Workplace injuries and illnesses for 2002. Bureau of Labor Statistics. Available at: http://www.bls.gov/news.release/pdf/osh.pdf. Accessed February 23, 2004.

[2] Newkirk WL. Occupational Health Services. Chicago: American Hospital Publishing, Inc; 1993. p. 1–10, 256.

[3] Systoc [computer program]. Version 7.1. Occupational Health Research. P.O. Box 900, 28 Research Drive, Skowhegan, ME, 04976. 2002.

[4] The U.S. Department of Labor. MSD as "injury or disorders of the muscles, nerves, tendons, joints, cartilage, and spinal column."

[5] U.S. Department of Labor. Lost work days. Bureau of Labor Statistics. Available at: http://www.bls.gov. Accessed November 2007.

[6] Fletcher, M. Over-exertion leading cause of comp claims: liberty business insurance. February 26, 2001.

[7] Reneman MF, Fokkens AS, Dijkstra PU, et al. Testing lifting capacity: validity of determining effort level by means of observation. Spine 2005;30(2): E40–6.

[8] Essential functions of the job CFR, specific to Title I of the American with Disabilities Act (29 CFR 1630).

[9] Normand J, Salyards SD, Mahoney JJ. An evaluation of pre-employment drug testing. Journal of Applied Psychology 1990;75(6):629–39.

[10] Mayer B, Hemphill G. Evaluation of urine creatinine as a marker to identify diluted specimens being evaluated for drugs of abuse. Clinical Chemistry 1991;38:1927–31.

[11] Newkirk WL, Ryder RA. Occupational Health Services. Chicago: American Hospital Publishing, Inc.; 1989. p. 6–13.

Further reading

Brassard M. The Memory Jogger Plus+. Methuen (MA): Goal/QPC; 1989.

Coffey R, Marszalek-Gaucher E. Transforming health care organizations: achieving and sustaining organizational excellence. San Francisco (CA): Jossey-Bass; 1990.

Health Care Advisory Board. TQM: 14. Tactics for improving the quality process. Washington, DC: The Advisory Board Company; 1992.

James BC. Quality management for health care delivery. Chicago: The Hospital Research and Education Trust; 1989.

La Dou J. Occupational medicine. East Norwalk (CT): Appleton and Lange; 1990.

Rom W, editor. Environmental and occupational medicine. Boston: Little Brown and Company; 1983.

Rom W, editor. Environmental and occupational medicine, 3rd edition. Philadelphia: Lippincott-Raven Publishers; 1998.

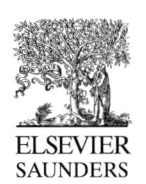

The Physician-Owned Orthotic and Durable Medical Equipment Service

William A. Bolesta, MS, BOC

Orthotic Consulting Services, PO Box 646, Hampstead, MD 21074, USA

In recent years, orthopedic practices have been forced to create internal ancillary profit centers to help compensate for escalating operating expenses. Increased professional liability premiums and health care costs, coupled with decreased reimbursements, have made the development of these ancillary centers a necessity.

Many practices engage in the more traditional ancillary profit centers: physician-owned MRI facilities, surgical centers, and physical therapy rehabilitation facilities. Although some orthopedic practices have created ancillary orthotic and durable-medical equipment (DME) divisions, most practices still outsource these services. Many of the practices that do operate these divisions fail to capitalize on their true revenue potential.

To establish the most profitable orthotic and DME division, physician practices need to assess and fully analyze all aspects of this ancillary service. Due diligence in evaluating key components of the division serves to expedite the creation of the service and to identify key components and issues that ultimately dictate the overall success of the center.

The marketplace offers several business models to help practices initiate and manage DME delivery. In particular, product manufacturers are developing programs to address the change from traditional outsourcing to physician-owned entities. Their intent is to assist the practice in developing and managing this ancillary. The design of many of these programs, however, tends to place the focus on sales of the manufacturer's product rather than on the practice's primary objective: maximum profitability.

Although many variables ultimately affect net revenue gains, practices need to identify hidden costs associated with many current program offerings. In addition, many common obstacles exist that seem to derail the creation of the division. Many administrators already are overburdened with daily business operations, and often the task of starting the process seems somewhat unrealistic.

Some practices may consider the challenges to establishing a DME ancillary service—Medicare regulations, certification and accreditation processes, coding and billing compliance, along with a host of other challenges—too great. A detailed, clearly defined Business plan can help most practices overcome these obstacles, streamline operations, and determine realistic revenue projections.

Practice assessment

Before initiating any form of ancillary service for orthotics and DME, a practice should perform a thorough assessment of its operations. Analysis of several factors will enable a practice to develop a detailed business plan and, ultimately, to maximize profitability.

Physician subspecialties/referral trends

Identifying physician specialties and how they directly relate to referral trends is an important first step in establishing a division. Certain specialties have higher referral patterns than others. Although training and prior education certainly affect physician referral trends, these trends often can be categorized into product groupings.

E-mail address: orthoticconsulting@comcast.net

0030-5898/08/$ - see front matter © 2008 Elsevier Inc. All rights reserved.
doi:10.1016/j.ocl.2007.09.003

orthopedic.theclinics.com

Individual preferences need to be evaluated to determine accurate usage volume, however.

Often, a practice may arrive at volume figures simply by multiplying the number of physicians by an estimate of per-physician revenue. This technique is not an accurate way to assess revenue potential or profitability, because an error in the estimate will be amplified by multiplication. Also, an accurate assessment must identify both off-the-shelf items and custom appliances. This survey also should include items currently obtained through local surgical centers and hospitals following surgery.

The evaluation process should resemble an interview process, with each physician associating diagnosis or Current Procedural Terminology (CPT) surgical codes with medically necessary equipment. The goal is both to identify treatment options for particular injuries and to educate physicians on new products and devices that may serve as an adjunctive treatment option and enhance the overall patient outcome. This process is a critical step in creating the foundation of the division, because referring volume will affect staffing, storage, and billing issues. The accuracy of this assessment also determines a practice's ability to gauge first-year revenue and profit.

Number of locations

Many practices, to compete for market share, expand their geographic coverage by establishing satellite locations. Although doing so increases patient referrals across a larger area, it also increases the amount of inventory required. Although inventory levels can be modified to meet the particular needs of the subspecialties within the group, it often is difficult to maintain control over the quantity and type of products stocked across a practice's various locations. This problem is especially significant for general orthopedic surgeons who see an array of conditions not specific to an extremity.

An accurate evaluation of physician subspecialties and product-referral trends can help tailor an initial stocking order for each location. After that, the practice must incorporate procedures to address ordering, designated staff involvement, and operational issues to standardize the billing for all locations.

Patient/surgical volume

Although physician referral trends in relation to diagnoses are critical, another key component is patient volume. The busier a practice is, the greater is the revenue potential for an orthotic and DME division. Physician education on treatment options and product alternatives can enhance revenue, but referring volume ultimately dictates profitability. Analyzing monthly patient volume and accurately assessing the surgical portion of business are crucial to accurate financial projections.

The type and number of surgical procedures performed will offer guidance in structuring the division. In addition, the practice must identify the DME prescribed, the prescription sequence, and the locations where patients obtain equipment.

Current staffing levels

Because administrators are forced to cross-train staff to minimize expenditures, the individuals on a physician support staff commonly perform a wide variety of tasks. The assessment process must take into account current staff obligations and anticipate the increased responsibilities involved in operating an orthotic and DME division.

The type of referral (custom or off-the-shelf) and associated volume will determine whether the current staff can absorb the increased duties and will determine if the staff has the related clinical experience to service the patients.

Product preferences/pricing

Many practices that operate an internal ancillary service or use an outsourcing model (stock and bill, on-site, or another model) rely on sales representatives to educate them on product selection. Often, a physician group decides to use a particular product or service because of an established relationship with a representative, rather than because of the qualities of the product itself.

Before establishing any orthotic and DME entity, the practice needs to evaluate product options and corresponding costs. Items should be evaluated with four main criteria as the baseline for selection: quality, cost, inventory control, and reimbursement.

Inventory storage and tracking

Inventory control is critical to the success of an orthotic and DME division, particularly in a practice with multiple locations. The practice needs to evaluate patient flow, storage space availability, and current billing operations within the framework of the office. Ideally, all products can be centralized with limited access, with designated staff responsible for monitoring the inventory.

The primary function of any inventory control system, regardless of the technology employed, is to monitor and regulate supply and demand. An efficient system should establish par levels, replenish items as dispensed, and accurately associate dispensed items with billing procedures to connect patient charges and reduce shrinkage. Physical inventory counts also are necessary to regulate and minimize shrinkage.

Space allocation

Most practices are under space constrictions or, at best, already have designated any future space to other uses. Depending on the type and volume of referrals, the practice may need to allocate designated space to accommodate the orthotic and DME division.

Most offices have an internal structure to expedite patient flow. The time between patient checkin to checkout is dictated, in large part, by examination-room occupancy. The last thing a practice wants to do is extend examination-room use for a patient being fitted for a brace, because doing so can increase waiting time for other patients or reduce overall patient volume. If possible, it is preferable to designate a specific location to treat brace referrals.

Designating a specific location is particularly important when servicing custom referrals. Even simple brace modifications can create dust, and many substances used within the area may need to be contained with proper ventilation and storage equipment. The extent of equipment needed, the size of the space, and the amount of storage will dictate the requirements for centralizing the division.

Billing processes

Before any discussion of product coding and fee schedules can take place, the practice needs to evaluate many elements contained within the current billing process of the practice. The key to any successful DME and orthotic operation is bridging the gap between the clinician and billing staff. Many of the operational issues can be addressed before the actual implementation phase, and doing so will help ensure the success of the center.

Depending on how the practice is structured, the surgical scheduler could play a key role in bringing efficiency to the process. Proper knowledge of coverage criteria, precertification guidelines, coding, and reimbursement ultimately affect the revenue of the division. Many DME products can be preauthorized at the time surgery is scheduled, greatly enhancing collections.

Often, existing practice management systems must be modified. For instance, encounter forms or super bills can be altered to accommodate the necessary coding for most of the appliances. Documentation procedures, especially for custom appliances, need to be written and incorporated into patient files, and forms need to be created to comply with regulations. It is critical to evaluate and establish these protocols before initiating the center.

Legal issues

All state and federal laws need to be reviewed as they pertain to a given location. Self-referral laws, Stark laws, and state laws could influence how the division is structured. Many states have licensure requirements for fitting certain classifications of appliances, and Medicare is proposing to mandate facility accreditation for orthotic and DME providers. It is advisable to confer with legal counsel and to appoint designated staff members to keep current with all upcoming changes and policies that may directly affect the ancillary division.

Payer information

A key part of the due diligence process is evaluating payer information. The practice administrator should obtain a breakdown of patient percentages as they relate to insurance carriers to determine the population demographics. Next, the billing department should evaluate each individual payer to determine the ability of the practice to perform orthotic and DME services.

In some cases, the practice simply can amend an existing contract to allow the group access. Others may require a separate application and credentialing process. Some carriers already have national contracts in place and do not allow physician groups to participate as DME providers.

Once a practice has identified carrier participation and practice eligibility and has cross-referenced the patient percentages, it should associate reimbursement rates for each carrier. Then, after all information has been analyzed, the practice can make an informed decision in relation to participation, requirements, and revenue projections.

Options for practices

Manufacturers have spent the past few years creating business models to assist practices in assuming control over DME. Practices should weigh the options provided by manufacturers carefully, however. Some models are geared more toward increasing product sales than toward creating an independent entity for the practice. Others make it virtually impossible for practices to capture fully the revenue that exists.

Many vendors now give some persons in their sales force the job title "consultant" in an effort to legitimize certain business models. For example, some offer "billing consultants" but as a company perform no third-party billing. The practice should take care to determine the qualifications of any consultant and the actual level of consultation it will receive.

Any practice should weigh carefully the revenue and profitability of any business model, taking care to determine whether that model is structured to provide the practice with the maximum revenue possible.

Inventory modules

One of the main attractions in evaluating ancillary DME business options involves inventory-control scanner modules. These systems offer sophisticated mobile scanner capabilities and can help regulate the inventory tracking issues most offices face.

Typically, these modules use bar codes to read data from product inventory, and some are adapting their formats to accommodate paperless electronic systems. The system can read bar codes from the existing manufacturer, or the vendor may create an internal bar code affixes either to the shelf or directly on the product.

The main functions of these systems are to monitor existing product levels, to incorporate a reorder mechanism to ensure adequate replenishment while minimizing PAR levels, and to associate dispensed items with accurate patient charges. Most systems on the market perform these functions, and several have additional features that can integrate billing functions.

Although the systems help navigate the tedious job of inventory management, many practices focus solely on inventory modules as the solution for establishing an orthotic and DME entity. In many cases, these vendors are product manufacturers, using the module as a means to sell product. Typically, most of the products offered are produced by the manufacturer, and the starting price may range from the wholesale price to 15% above wholesale, depending whether product is initially stored on consignment. In addition, the inventory module may carry a license fee and monthly usage charges, in addition to the cost of the scanners.

Thus there are significant drawbacks to incorporating an inventory module offered by a manufacturer. First, it can curtail product selection severely and perhaps even compromise product quality. Second, it can involve higher-than-necessary product costs. Third, it constitutes only one element of a full-fledged orthotic and DME division.

Inventory control is important, but it is only one of many important areas that need to be addressed when evaluating and developing an orthotic and DME division.

Physicians should use caution when evaluating the pros and cons of each service and should evaluate and compare options thoroughly before investing in a program.

Combination stock-and-bill/billing for select items

In another model, a vendor offers a modified billing program aimed at generating ancillary revenue for a practice. Under this arrangement, a manufacturer allows the practice to bill independently for select items, while the manufacturer maintains a stock-and-bill format for the remaining items.

Although this model can increase revenue for the practice, it still limits the revenue potential that exists for the practice. In addition, the product designated for sale by the practice may carry a higher price than the practice could negotiate separately.

Although the lower-cost items represent smaller gross revenue, the collective volume associated with dispensing all items will yield a far better return than merely concentrating on select items.

In addition, a practice still must carry the same additional overhead expenses, with possible additional expenses that accompany increased volume. Furthermore, under this arrangement, the practice typically does not capture revenue from custom bracing and DME items that can enhance revenue significantly.

Most practices considering this model would benefit from exploring the possibility of creating an entire practice-operated division instead of resorting to half-measures.

Shared revenue

The goal of the shared-revenue model is to help orthopedic practices capture revenue through the development of a modified internal entity. Under this model, a vendor supplies a clinician to act as the designated staff member in charge of fitting appliances and monitoring inventory.

The vendor bills the item, using the practice's provider numbers, and then deducts costs from receivables to cover clinician salary expenses, billing fees, and cost of goods sold. The remaining profit is then split based on a predetermined percentage.

There are disadvantages to this arrangement aside from the Medicare regulatory issues. One of the biggest is that the practice's final profit is a fraction of what it would be if the practice developed an independent division. Most practices simply can add the associated product charges to the super bill, eliminating any added billing fees associated with the service. In addition, the vendor product charges usually are inflated, and the designated staff is not the practice's employee and cannot be cross-trained to support daily office functions.

Any practice should determine the potential of the shared-revenue model on its own independent revenue projection and not rely on a vendor's projection that may be simplistic or inaccurate. Often, a practice will find that creating its own division makes better fiscal sense than forfeiting a large percentage of profit. In most instances, an arrangement to work with another company to establish an orthotic and DME division should be based on fixed fees, independent of revenue.

Existing entity

Some practices have already implemented an internal entity and are reaping the rewards of this relatively recent ancillary profit center. Most practices that have created this division remain marginally profitable at best, however, and others lack true auditing mechanisms to identify accurate revenue projections.

The problem with most facilities that have created this entity is that the three main components of the division act independently and lack the critical communication processes required to monitor the entity. Clinical, billing, and collections all need to be involved in the entire process, or at least in the set-up, to interact and transmit information for analysis.

The practice needs to have an internal auditor who will monitor associated charges and coding to ensure compliance and accurate processing. If payments are denied because of issues relating to coding or classification of injury, the information needs to be forwarded back to the clinician. Does the practice know the shrinkage percentages in relation to cost of goods sold? Does the practice identify payer trends and physician-referral trends or monitor product evaluations that may enhance revenue or quality?

In many cases, clinicians hired to perform the actual job description are not focused on business and may not confer regularly with physicians. Is there an incentive for the hired clinician to increase business, and is the clinician knowledgeable enough to act as the business liaison for the division? Although most practices have the right instinct, they fail to maximize the potential of their division. Often, a full assessment can redefine objectives that will lead to increased opportunities.

Creating or enhancing the division

After a full practice assessment has been completed, and a thorough evaluation of service offerings has been performed, the practice needs to create the division. The assessment will provide critical information that defines objectives and lays the foundation for the development of a strategic plan and for implementing that plan in an orderly sequence and in a timely fashion.

Product selection

One of the first steps in initiating an orthotic and DME program is to identify and confirm the product selection process. Practices should begin by forming a small committee to evaluate options, beginning with items that the practice currently uses and is familiar with. The next step is to research several additional manufacturers' options in relation to body part and to obtain product samples for comparison. Approximately two to five samples should be obtained for each comparison.

The evaluation process should identify and compare the four main components involved in final product selection: the quality of product, the cost of the item, its reimbursement value in relation to CPT coding, and the ability of the item to assist with inventory control.

Quality

Product quality should be one of the main factors in product comparison. The products dispensed and billed within an office are a direct reflection of the practice's reputation. Product failures and breakdowns that occur more frequently in lower-quality products put future referrals at risk. The product should maintain an appealing image, and the materials should be constructed in a durable manner with adequate warranty periods. Finally, members of the committee should try on the products to get a firsthand idea of the quality and feel of the appliances.

Cost

Cost is always a concern when deciding on product. Most manufacturers, to stay competitive, establish similar pricing structures on related products. Many manufacturers will discount, depending on referring volume. Some manufacturers have better profit margins than others on select items that may influence the ability to discount. One should organize the products in relation to cost and then return to the initial quality selection process. In most cases, the higher-priced items are also the higher-quality products. The goal is to find the medium range that will suffice for price but not lower standards in terms of quality selection.

Coding

Most items are associated with CPT codes for reimbursement. These codes are descriptive but often are very general. Products should be associated with the most accurate coding description, without cost of the product influencing the decision. New codes are continually being modified, deleted, and added. Many manufacturers cater product design to accommodate these new coding descriptions. The provider, however, must bypass manufacturer recommendations and thoroughly review each product to assign appropriate CPT codes. It is ultimately the provider who is responsible for coding accuracy, not the manufacturer.

Some manufacturers submit appliances for Medicare approval and request a specific CPT code for the product, eliminating any guesswork for providers. Most manufacturers, however, do not follow this process because it may put them at risk of having the product delegated to a coding level that carries a lower reimbursement level than they believe is accurate.

Practices can evaluate product options and related CPT coding to explore possible product alternatives. Generally, payers associate diagnosis codes with CPT codes for reimbursement. Payers will not pay for a knee brace if the primary diagnosis is located in the ankle. It may be possible, however, to supplement or upgrade certain appliances to increase reimbursement.

For example, practices may choose from a vast array of off-the-shelf spinal orthoses, from simple elastic corsets to thoracolumbar spinal orthoses. Many products have been designed specifically to accommodate the continually evolving coding descriptions. Physicians need to evaluate specific design, function, and indications for use and then compare existing product selections. Often physicians are unaware of new options, and these alternative selections can enhance revenue dramatically. The physician obviously needs to retain ethical compliance and not prescribe items that are not medically indicated. Careful examination of potential upgrades, however, can improve patient outcomes and increase revenue projections.

Universal fitting appliances

Many manufacturers also are trying to develop items that are inventory-control conscious. Providing universal fitting appliances that do not lower the quality of the product or affect function can reduce inventory levels by as much as 80%. This consideration is especially important when practices have multiple satellite locations. The selection committee should include product options that address this important feature.

Preoperative protocols and referral trends

After the selection process is completed, the next step involves developing preoperative protocols and defining specific physician-referral trends in relation to diagnosis and CPT codes. This process should be performed with product groupings associated with specific procedures. For instance, an anterior cruciate ligament surgery should include product options such a crutches, a postoperative brace, cold therapy, functional braces, and possibly continuous passive motion (CPM) devices. Although not dictating protocol, the intent is to create a definitive treatment plan and coordinate most services preoperatively to capture the referrals.

This concept virtually eliminates any decision making for the physicians once the protocol is implemented. The process streamlines operations, enhances patient care and compliance, reduces associated expenses at the surgical locations, and enhances revenue for the practice.

This protocol should be developed for every surgical procedure that may require the use of a medically necessary piece of equipment. Although this process focuses only on the surgical portion of business, it represents a major segment of the typical practice's overall business.

After the preoperative phase is complete, the focus should move to treatment options for the more common office-visit referrals. For example, fracture care and treatment for sprains and overuse injuries can add significantly to the bottom line.

Staffing

Depending on the level and scope of referrals, the practice has to evaluate the current staffing demands in relation to anticipated added responsibilities. Referral patterns will dictate the level of experience needed to service patients.

If a practice prescribes a high number of custom appliances, it may elect to hire an orthotist. If the custom referrals typically involve the foot, perhaps the practice would opt to hire a pedorthist. If associated custom referrals are relatively low, it may make sense either to outsource that segment of business or to train one of the existing or new staff members to accommodate only that segment of referral. Referring volume certainly will dictate the type and scope of services that need to be created.

Inventory levels and storage

As soon as staffing and referring volume have been analyzed, the practice needs to begin structuring space allocation and inventory control options. Centralizing inventory is crucial in minimizing shrinkage, and designating staff to oversee the profit center will help monitor the division and make it more efficient and productive.

Although most practice management systems have inventory features, most of these software packages are limited in their functional capabilities. Facilities should try to incorporate some sort of software or scanner system that can assist with tracking and ordering products. Physical inventory levels still need to be taken to monitor shrinkage, and practices must create policies to address product disbursement for indigent patients. No inventory system, regardless of the technology, will work unless items that are dispensed are recorded or scanned, even if the practice elects not to charge for a particular item. Because most systems are established to replenish product as used, items need to be recorded when dispensed.

It is advisable to coordinate a training and education session on the use of the system and to set policies and procedures before initiating any format. PAR levels need to be determined based on usage trends or referral reports and incorporated into the module. Initial starting inventory levels need to be monitored after start-up, with physical inventory counts taken monthly to evaluate shrinkage. The initial inventory PAR levels can be modified after several months based on evaluation of actual usage patterns.

Although the design of the designated space for product storage may seem unimportant, it is crucial to structure it to meet anticipated demands. Inventory storage, if incorporated within the existing office, must provide ample space to accommodate supplies. If serving several locations, inventory should be centralized to reduce the quantity of on-hand inventory necessary to service a practice. The practice should limit access to inventory and delegate certain staff to oversee the entire division.

A designated inventory location outside the main office but within the same building can influence the dramatically scope of products offered. Depending on the type of appliances referred, the new location can be designed to resemble a separate orthotic and prosthetic facility. Having a separate waiting area, examination rooms, and laboratory area to make modifications can expand the potential of the ancillary center. The separate location then can apply for facility accreditation, as long as the design meets the requirements of the application process. By following this path, the practice can distinguish itself as a premier provider and meet potential regulation requirements in the future.

Inventory module

The next step in establishing a viable orthotic and DME division involves incorporating an inventory module into the practice's operations.

Most inventory modules can create multiple bar code labels, and most manufacturers already assign triplicate labels to all product boxes. Clinicians affix either the manufacturer's label or the custom label to the charge ticket. All forms then can be gathered at the end of the day and scanned at one centrally located site that has a tethered scanner and personal computer. Another option is to use mobile scanners that eliminate the need to tally forms, but an additional cost is associated with the mobile devices.

Custom-creating the labels can have certain benefits, especially if the program enables the practice to add associated CPT codes and charges to the label. This information will help the billing department assign corresponding charges. Some inventory modules may have the ability to integrate with the existing management software, which can assign these features. An inventory module system also provides the division with reporting and tracking capabilities, monitors shrinkage, and assures products dispensed are in fact billed correctly.

The reporting capabilities of the inventory module enable a practice to evaluate quickly and easily physician referral trends, usage patterns within locations, product profitability, and cost of goods sold in relation to net revenue.

Staff training

The level and scope of staff training, excluding the use of the inventory system, will depend on the type of products dispensed. Practices can send designated staff to specific courses or related orthotic and bracing seminars to maximize capturing of physician referrals.

If new full-time employees are required because of the demands of currently assigned responsibilities or the limited experience of existing staff, the practice can hire accordingly.

Expanding products and services

Although initially a division may concentrate primarily on off-the-shelf and custom orthotic appliances, it also can expand into the DME sector. Items such as cold therapy, ambulatory aids, CPM, and bone-growth stimulators can be integrated into a practice's overall service offering.

Many of these items typically are provided through a surgical center or hospital following surgery. Some items traditionally are noncovered, so they usually are distributed through these channels to eliminate or reduce the patient's financial responsibility. If a practice owns a surgical center and also provides these items, however, the practice is losing significant revenue. The items can be issued through preoperative protocols and billed before surgery. Doing so reduces expenses associated with the fixed reimbursements obtained within the surgical centers and generates revenue through billings applied to the division.

Some cold therapy devices are covered, and select units can be billed as compression devices if they offer sequential compression as part of the unit. These devices should be sent to insurance carriers as a payer survey to obtain coverage criteria in writing and payment options for each before they are implemented into the division. At minimum, practices can rent the devices or charge cash for the units. If the benefits are explained to a patient before dispensing the device, the patient can make an educated decision about purchasing or renting the device. This procedure eliminates any confusion and informs the patient in advance of options and coverage.

Typically, bone-growth stimulators are referred to designated manufacturer's representatives for both servicing and billing. Select companies, however, do allow practices to purchase and bill for the devices separately. Practices need to be educated on pertinent billing and coverage criteria before initiating any billing program, because these devices are expensive. Although typically used for non-union fractures, they also can be authorized as an adjunct to many two-level spinal fusions. This way, the devices can be obtained and authorized before surgery, eliminating any doubt about coverage criteria.

CPM machines are becoming less indicated for anterior cruciate repairs, mainly because of advanced surgical procedures and accelerated rehabilitation. Many physicians, however, still prescribe CPM machines for use following total knee replacement. Although practices are not allowed to provide these devices for Medicare patients, who may amount to 40% to 60% of the referred volume for a typical practice, they can provide these devices for other payers. Depending on the associated volume and individual referral trends of the group, CPM machines may be another option for the practice to generate revenue.

The main goal is to identify referral trends and then to design and implement a program that will capture the majority of appliances prescribed. After the program is operational, the goal should be to analyze referral trends and enhance the volume of referrals through physician education. Capturing all types of referrals from the orthotic and DME entities will maximize the division's revenue.

Overcoming common obstacles

Practice administrators face numerous challenges today in balancing the responsibilities associated with running an orthopedic practice. In addition to overseeing all aspects of daily operations, administrators have the added burden of trying to maintain profitability in an environment of decreasing reimbursement.

Many practices today turn to technological improvements that bring efficiency to operations: electronic medical record systems, digital imaging, and practice management software. These programs can place significant time constraints on administrative staff and on the entire practice. Launching these new programs can drain resources, forcing administrators to prioritize their efforts. Nonetheless, practices view these systems as essential in consolidating and streamlining operations. Although they carry an initial capital expenditure, the cost savings can be recouped relatively quickly, and functional outcomes can be defined appropriately. In general, however, these systems tend to reduce expenditures rather than generate revenue.

An ancillary orthotic division is different: it can significantly enhance or generate revenue. Often, however, practices do not define clearly a timeframe for initial set-up, implementation, and completion of the process. Without proper due diligence and careful analysis of the key aspects that define profitability, a practice will be unable to arrive at accurate projections and return on investment. Administrators should research options, perform reference checks, and thoroughly assess the practice before initiating any service.

As in any successful business, creating a detailed operational plan with specific objectives and defined parameters will help to ensure the success of the entity.

Meeting the challenges in the future

Although creating a structurally sound division certainly will enhance revenue, practices need to prepare for challenges in the future that will impact profitability. Health Insurance Portability and Accountability Act regulations, although much needed, placed a burden on practices to adopt policies to meet requirements. These regulations increase time and staff demands, ultimately placing added expenses on the practice. Similarly, practices will need to invest time and resources to comply with future requirements in the Orthotic and Prosthetic and DME sector.

Staff certification and facility accreditation requirements will standardize care, but at a cost. Insurance reimbursements are continually decreasing, and even Medicare is implementing competitive bidding in certain states in 2007 that will reduce reimbursement on select off-the-shelf items, perhaps by 20% or more. These issues will affect the overall net revenue within each division and reinforce the need to develop a thorough ancillary center that targets capturing all referrals.

Summary

Although orthotic and ancillary profit centers can enhance the overall revenue stream for orthopedic practices, administrators need to analyze pertinent information before developing the entity. The ability of the practice to navigate successfully through the obstacles of creating the division, and through future challenges, ultimately will define profitability within the center.

Although many programs are aimed at assisting with this venture, practices need to use caution when evaluating these programs. Many of these offerings may not deliver the promised profitability for the practices, but a practice will know for certain only if it engages in a rigorous independent assessment . Increased product costs, the inability to create programs that capture all referrals, and future requirements can leave practices at a loss when a final profitability assessment is performed.

Practices that assess and incorporate sound business polices in developing the entity, monitor its progression, and strive to enhance the overall offerings within the division will derive the most profitability. By following a structured plan, practices can maximize revenue potential and improve patient satisfaction and outcomes.

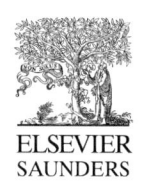

Medical Opinions: The Physician-Owned Independent Medical Examination Company

Stephanie Rozman, Victoria L. Rude, Judy Polasky

6800 France Avenue S., Suite 300, Edina, MN 55435, USA

Overview of the independent medical examination industry

It is common in an injury claim situation for a legitimate dispute to exist about the cause of the condition at issue or the nature and extent of the injury or disability. Reasonable minds can and do differ about these issues. The trier of fact must resolve the dispute, and independent medical examinations (IMEs) play an essential role in this process. IMEs help to determine compensability, the necessity of treatment and type of treatment, the extent of disability, and the evaluation of permanent impairment and/or loss of earning capacity.

The actual beginning of the IME industry is somewhat obscure. It was not until the postwar era, the late 1940s and 1950s, that the precursor of modern IMEs came into being. In many states IMEs were not referred to as "independent medical examinations," but rather as "insurance medical examinations" or, in workers' compensation terms, "examinations by the employer's physicians." Initially, insurance-related medical examinations were performed by individual physicians in their own clinics. Although the term "IME" had replaced other terms during the 1960s, it did not come into common usage until the birth of the IME companies.

In the late 1960s and early 1970s there was a fundamental shift in the industry with the formation of IME companies. As state workers' compensation systems evolved, and with many states changing to no-fault systems for motor vehicle accident injuries, the IME industry changed and grew. The 1970s and 1980s gave rise to an increasing intolerance for insurance fraud. Added to this intolerance was concern from another angle, that of ensuring that the claimants received appropriate medical treatment and that the insurance/legal systems did not go unchecked. In the 1990s, based on a heightened sense of professionalism, the industry came to realize the advantages to be gained by raising its own standards. IME companies sought ways to achieve a greater level of legitimacy.

One of the issues that long vexed the IME industry was the questionable relationship between the IME industry and insurers. Time and again critics ask how IME facilities can guarantee impartial examinations when the insurer is paying the bill, may be looking to minimize its exposure, and may take its business elsewhere. During the 1990s the IME industry itself seemed to recognize the ethical dilemma of trying to render medical opinions favorable only to the insurer. Whatever actual or imagined pressure IME physicians once may have felt to opine in favor of the insurer has lessened as IME companies redefined themselves. Because of this shift in philosophy, the marketability of physicians whose reports are without basis has waned tremendously.

The authors of this article works for a physician-owned IME company. Their experience has revealed that this company, owned by credible physicians with thriving clinical practices, seems to have an ethical advantage. These physicians are primarily treating physicians who view participation in the medicolegal process in keeping with medicine's greater mission of helping to relieve suffering. They serve their communities with their participation. The commercial rewards are a secondary byproduct. It is as possible to see adverse (to the insurance carriers) medical opinions as favorable ones. It all depends on the medical rationale.

E-mail address: stephanier@evalumed.com (S. Rozman)

Critical factors to assess when considering start up of an independent medical examination company

By understanding his or her professional goals and then thoroughly analyzing the industry and its players, applicable laws, and the overall cost versus benefits, a physician can assess the feasibility of establishing his or her own IME company and the commitment that comes with success. Physicians interested in participating in the IME industry should determine the model that is right for their business, talents, and expertise. Even an occasional IME may round out one's practice or provide a different insight into the challenging world of health care delivery.

Opportunity costs

The potential opportunity cost associated with owning an IME company is the loss of revenue relative to the physician's clinical practice. There are only 24 hours in a day, and time from the clinical practice will need to be reallocated to the IME aspects of the business: conducting examinations, reviewing records, writing reports, offering testimony, and supervising and/or consulting the overall operation.

Regulatory environment

Several general requirements are universal, but the procedural rules governing IMEs vary among federal and state jurisdictions for tort cases as well as for cases involving statutory claims such as workers' compensation.

It is of the utmost importance to consult with an attorney to seek advice regarding the applicable state laws with regard to possible statutory provisions governing IMEs in general, statutes governing various insurance coverages (eg, workers' compensation and automobile no-fault statutes) and the parameters or limitations on performing IMEs in the state or states in which business will be conducted. When present, these statutory provisions generally provide rules regarding who can attend an IME in terms of third parties, the location of the IME, who is entitled to a copy of the IME report, the billing of the IME and other services, and the timing of an IME. All of these considerations are important, and many company policies are likely to be based on applicable state laws.

Competitor analysis

The IME industry is a service-driven industry with very little barrier to entry. Any improvement that can be made in the services currently provided in the local marketplace may provide a competitive advantage but also may be the cause of the company's demise if excellent service ultimately cannot be delivered. An analysis of the competition's strengths and weaknesses, looking for opportunities to improve on service, is well worth the effort. How can service be delivered better?

In an underserved market, business may come quite quickly as word spreads that a new service provider is in the area. In a crowded field, however, a newly formed company may need to be more aggressive with its marketing efforts. Business volume will take time to build.

A competitive advantage comes with finding a middle ground, a balance between stability and change (Box 1).

Financial needs

Operating capital is necessary to seed development and to sustain the business as it grows. People, office space, equipment, and marketing expenses are just a few of the cost centers that may require investment before revenues can be experienced.

Strategic planning

Strategy for a successful IME company has everything to do with

1. Knowing the customers: Who are they? What are their needs?
2. Putting together a panel of credible physicians
3. Informing potential clients about the panel of medical experts (Fig. 1)

Customers

Who are the customers/clients? Their organizational type and job titles can vary.

Box 1. Factors encouraging stability and change

To encourage stability
Develop home-grown management
Be clear about the core ideology
Create family-like atmosphere

To encourage change
Set goals high
Try a lot and keep what works
Good enough never is

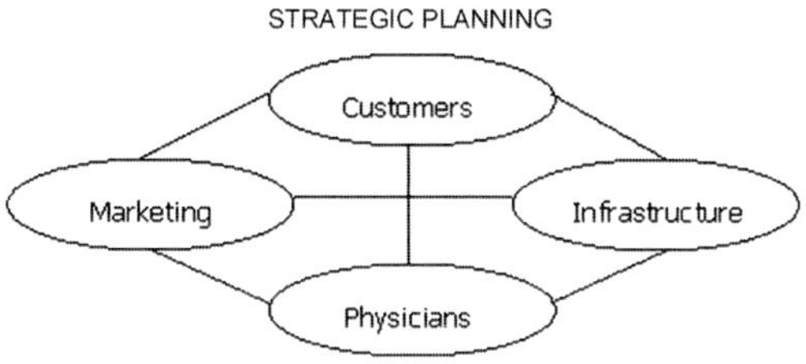

Fig. 1. Strategic planning

Organization type
- Insurance carrier
- Third-party claims administrator
- Self-insured employer
- Government
- Legal practice

Job titles
- Adjuster
- Claims supervisor
- Claims executive
- Nurse case manager
- Attorney

Some of their needs are common; others are influenced by geographic considerations.

Common needs

There are common needs that many clients share. Clients are looking for strong physician credentials, specialization and expertise appropriate to each case, awareness of relevant laws and terminology, thorough, well-reasoned reports that enable claims and/or court decisions to be made, and a willingness to back up reports effectively with depositions and testimony, if required.

Geographic needs

Geographic needs vary from client to client, and even within one organization there may be claims personnel who handle different territories. Claims handlers, nurse case managers, or attorneys managing local claims may deal with one or only a few cities. They will know IME doctors by experience and reputation. Claims handlers managing regional claims usually deal throughout one or several states. They know some doctors by experience and reputation but use IME vendors to fill in gaps relative to referral needs. Claims handlers managing national claims deal with cases anywhere in the country. They know only a few physicians and rely heavily on IME companies to tap into reputable physician networks. As the IME company grows, expanding the physician panel to include reputable physicians around the country allows the company to meet the breadth of loyal customers' needs.

Provider panel

Recruiting a panel of medical experts will translate into a solid physician network with depth and a variety of specialties represented. This network is the foundation of a successful IME company. Certainly many injuries seen in the medicolegal context are orthopedic injuries, but experts in neurology, occupational medicine, psychiatry, pulmonology, internal medicine, and infectious disease also are frequently consulted in the medicolegal context. Also, orthopedic surgeons who subspecialize in spine surgery or hand surgery are invaluable. If a community does not provide a sufficient representation of these specialties, and specifically a sufficient number of orthopedic surgeons, nearby communities may.

The IME industry seeks physicians who are board certified and active in their practice. Because an IME is a tool often used in the court of law, a physician's curriculum vitae and reputation sometimes are questioned. Leading IME physicians are open-minded, valued for their medical expertise and knowledge, and skilled at presenting their medical opinions in a thorough and compelling manner.

Physicians who are well respected within their community and among their peers have the greatest inherent credibility in the medicolegal setting. Credentials and professional qualifications should be verified before affiliating with any physician within the network. There are many credentialing companies that provide these services for a fairly nominal fee. The time saved is well worth the cost. If the company is fortunate, the affiliated physicians will have some degree of IME experience. Many physicians, however, will not and will need to be provided with the necessary tools to be successful and to contribute to the overall success of the company. It is helpful to work with a local law firm to develop a training program or training manual for physicians that addresses the legal concepts and terminology of the applicable state laws governing the types of cases that will be encountered, as well as tips or guidelines for deposition preparation and deposition testimony. An outline of the legal process and definition of legal terms for various types of claims is helpful to provide an overview and framework of how the system works. There also are national training programs with certifications that physicians can attain with regard to performing IMEs.

At the time of affiliation, the company will need to outline expectations clearly to each physician in terms of the services he or she provides. It is important to address issues such as the overall process from the scheduling of the appointment to billing, expected turnaround time for reports, the elements of a comprehensive IME report, client expectations with regard to report quality and accessibility, and compensation for services. If expectations are not set forth from the beginning, and bad habits are created, the company will have difficulty later.

As the IME company grows, physician recruitment will be an ongoing process driven by client needs, client recommendations, and trends in insurance claims as well as litigation.

Sales and marketing

Getting the message out to the clients about the panel of medical experts is achieved through a viable marketing plan. Leading IME companies understand the value and need for committed and continuous marketing and sales efforts and therefore employ experienced staff to acquire clients and to ensure that their needs are met. These efforts foster long-term client relationships. This department also requires the assistance of promotional tools, such as Websites, collateral material, and promotional events that are created internally or with help of outside marketing experts. Understanding and communicating how the IME company differs from others will help position it in the marketplace.

Assessing goals and objectives, the marketing mix, and budget limitations to come up with a marketing plan is key. Product, price, place, and promotion make up the marketing mix (Box 2).

Product

Medical opinions are sought when the worlds of medicine and law intersect. The opinions can be packaged in a number of different ways. This packaging is, of course, client driven and based on the client's needs. Successful IME companies offer an expansive array of ways to package the expert opinions, including, but not limited to, IMEs, second opinions, third-party evaluations, disability examinations, advice-to-pay evaluations, return-to-work evaluations, record reviews, peer reviews, and diagnostic film reviews. These presentations correlate with laws surrounding workers' compensation, automobile no-fault, automobile tort, general liability, product liability, long- and short-term disability, and the Family Medical Leave Act.

The IME industry and its primary clients, insurance companies and legal firms, function within a time-sensitive and demanding environment in which exceptional service is expected. In fact, if a commitment to service cannot be created and maintained, entering the industry will be a fruitless endeavor. One should be prepared for

---

Box 2. The marketing mix

Product
- The IME product is a mix of product and service:
High-quality IME reports, thorough and well reasoned
Commitment to excellent customer service

Price
- Pricing is one component of the competitive offering.
- Understanding current pricing in the marketserved is important: what is customary varies around the country.
- The right price depends on goals, objectives, and the regulatory environment.

Place
- Single versus multiple office locations
- Travel to other cities
- Leasing space for IMEs or working with other medical providers who facilitate IMEs at their locations

Promotion
- Advertising in legal/claims publications
- IME directories
- Network participation
- Ongoing marketing/sales staff client relations
- Participation in professional organizations (American Board of Independent Medical Examiners, American Academy of Disability Evaluating Physicians)
- Speaking engagements
- Trade shows
- Interactive Website

a client-driven culture in which both proactive and reactive activities are required on a daily basis. Additionally, all IME companies typically employ servicing representatives who acquire and maintain new clients through various customer-service techniques. Clients are easily persuaded to try a new vendor for their medical/legal services solely by a poor service experience. This tendency is good news for companies that offer consistently great service but is bad news for those that lack this commitment and expertise.

Looking to the competitors and potential customers in the market place to establish service guidelines for the company is helpful. What is the standard turnaround time for an IME report in the community? What are the needs and expectations of the customers? Based on this information, reasonable guidelines for delivering more than is promised are set initially. The list of customer needs is growing ever longer, and just one service-related issue could cost a company a customer for life.

Price

The accounting department will need to be familiar with industry billing practices and state-mandated billing guidelines to set pricing policies.

Place

How accessible are the physicians on the company's provider panel? Applicable state laws may place parameters (eg, a mileage radius from the home of the examinee) on the location of the IME. If the locations for examinations are not offered within a major population center, being outside the legal travel distance for most potential examinees can be a problem. The company's primary facility should be located easily and in a larger city or more populated area. Several service sites may be required for overall accessibility and convenience. Many clinics will allow outside physicians to perform IMEs at their clinic sites for a nominal fee. Any examination facility should be easy to locate and access and should provide plenty of parking.

Promotion

Visibility in the market is crucial. Brochures and other materials as well as a Website and on-line access are standard marketing tools.

Organizational design of an IME company

Active physicians in private clinical practice do not have the time necessary to devote to make an IME company a success. It is beneficial to hire someone who shares the vision and has extensive experience in the insurance industry as well as sales or marketing experience. This individual would need to be familiar with the information systems of the company and its overall operating procedures, including the various functions of each department.

Systems

Systems and process models that optimize efficiency and quality are necessary to compete in the market place.

Systems/information technology

Although simple manual systems can be used to coordinate the IME process, today's leading IME companies have established extensive scheduling and information technology systems to track and understand the dynamics of their growing business, thus serving their clients quickly and efficiently.

Many IME companies have created custom-designed computer operating systems tailored to fit their specific needs in tracking, storing, and organizing information as well as reporting capabilities. This approach certainly provides the greatest flexibility in making changes and updating the system as ways to improve upon it are learned. There is also computer software available for IME companies.

Dictation systems

Digital dictation and digital speech standard dictation are the prevalent types of dictation in the industry. Digital dictation usually requires that the physician call an 800 number and dictate over the telephone. The company may provide its own digital service or may outsource dictation, which is one way to limit overhead start-up costs. Throughout the United States there are companies that specialize in transcribing medical dictation for as little as 10 cents per line. Physicians call an 800 number and dictate their reports. The turnaround time with these services is usually 24 hours. Digital speech standard dictation uses a handheld digital recorder that stores the physician's dictation as an audio file on a small disk within the recorder. The files can be downloaded to a computer and e-mailed to the IME company. Even if physician dictation is outsourced, the company will need in-house staff to handle any other transcription needs that may arise. A medical transcription background is imperative.

Records management

The computer operating system chosen for the company can help store and organize medical records as well as provide on-line access. In a paperless system, on-line access to chart items such as the client's cover letter or background letter is especially critical to the quality assurance review process provided by the quality assurance department.

Staff and skill sets

Staffing models that optimize efficiency and quality are invaluable to a successful IME company.

Current clinical staff may not have the expertise, knowledge, or available time required to support the needs of an IME company. The company will need to assess both staff qualifications and what portion of any given work day can be committed to the new company. All aspects need to be considered, including scheduling, medical record gathering/organization, transcription, quality assurance, and billing and accounting (Fig. 2).

Scheduling

Often considered "inside sales," the scheduling department is on the front line, and first impressions are crucial. Scheduling usually is the client's first real interaction with the company. It is imperative that the schedulers understand the physician network intimately, including such details as the physicians' specialties, subspecialties, IME schedules, and locations. It also is helpful for scheduling to know clinic affiliations, report quality, and style. A scheduler who has worked previously with physicians in the context of a busy clinical setting is a good match for the fast-paced environment of the scheduling department where attention to every detail matters. Because of the service-driven nature of the industry, staff should be added to this department proactively in anticipation of growth rather than in hindsight. If the scheduling department cannot keep up with the incoming calls, clients who get a busy signal or who have been kept on hold will hang up and call a competitor. Also, some clients demand more time from a scheduler than other clients do, and adequate staffing allows the department to address the needs of all clients, ultimately resulting in better customer service overall.

The scheduling department staff must be skilled at identifying the physician who best matches the client's needs. The scheduling staff is responsible for confirming all aspects of the physician's time, including initially establishing the physician's availability, scheduling of IME appointments, rescheduling, providing written confirmations to clients and examinees, and noting cancellations as they occur.

Medical records

This department tracks receipt of and prepares all medical records and diagnostics for delivery to the physician before the scheduled IME. Specific chart preparation is designated by the physician

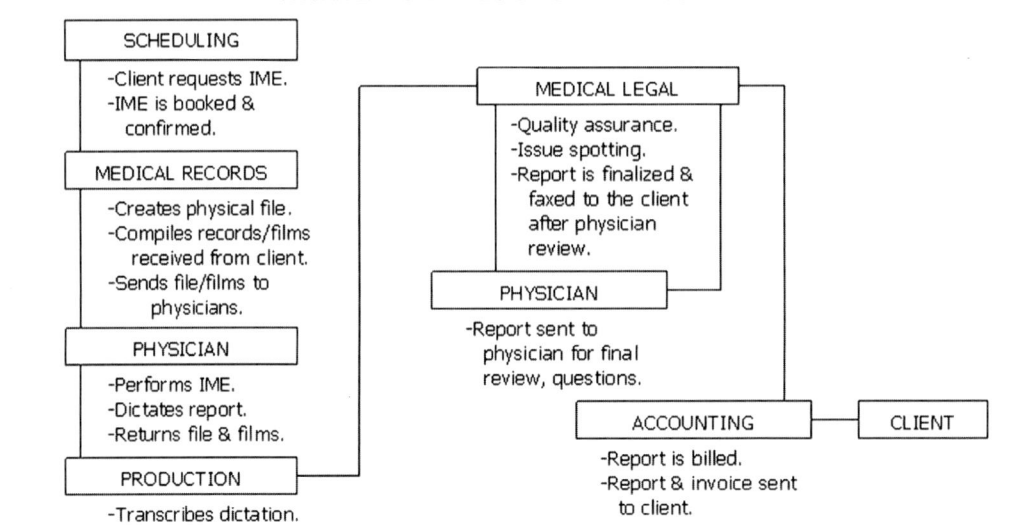

Fig. 2. Organizational design of an IME company

and may include tabbing operative and diagnostic reports or organizing records in chronologic order by provider or facility. A medical records background for potential staff is useful but not critical.

Clients usually are responsible for obtaining the medical records and other documentation. Clients are encouraged to provide medical records at least 1 week before the evaluation is scheduled. Organization of the records is also encouraged. Whenever an IME is scheduled, the medical records department will coordinate all medical record information relevant to the services requested. Once received from the client, records are forwarded to the correct physician in a timely manner, before the scheduled service date.

Medical records management as a service to the physicians is key, because the medical record documentation is the investigative "paper trail." An analysis of the records will help determine the validity of the claimant's injuries.

Transcription

Regardless of dictation preferences, (ie, voice recorder, written notes, electronic files), a physician-owned IME company will need trained medical transcriptionists who transcribe dictation or reformat written material and who track deadline dates to ensure timely completion and delivery to the client.

Quality assurance

Quality assurance departments were nonexistent in the IME industry before the 1980s. Now, based on a heightened sense of professionalism and the industry's realization of the advantages to be gained by raising its own standards, these departments have become a prominent feature of the larger IME companies. Nurse case consultants were the first to staff these quality assurance departments. They worked with the physicians on the technical/legal aspects of their reports, thereby pushing the physicians to produce thorough and well-reasoned reports.

The quality assurance staff is responsible for reviewing the rough-draft IME reports generated by physicians in a medicolegal context. The goals of this review process are to ensure a grammatically correct report that is formatted in a user-friendly way. The staff in this department can assist physicians in issuing thorough reports with sound reasoning that respond to the client's specific interrogatories.

Challenging legal concepts and issues are part of the IME arena and include

- Absence of relevant records
- Apportionment
- Causality
- Impairment ratings
- Identifying symptom magnification and malingering
- Maintaining independence
- State laws and terminology

Several general principles are universal, but the rules governing IMEs vary among federal and state jurisdictions for tort cases as well as for cases involving statutory claims such as workers' compensation. The volume of claims is heavy. It is essential to be concise but to provide adequate foundation for opinions. For example, many workers' compensation hearings are a mere 15 minutes long.

Staff in this department can assist IME physicians in

- Streamlining reports
- Meeting the medicolegal challenges
- Meeting the legal standard in a work comp, auto or liability case
- Eliminating inconsistency

To staff this department, the best-qualified individuals have a medical, legal, or insurance claims background. A well-rounded team would consist of an attorney, a nurse, and a claims adjuster, encompassing all three areas of expertise.

Accounting and finance

The company will need individuals familiar with industry billing practices and state-mandated billing guidelines to handle physician payroll and set pricing policies. This department also is responsible for budget planning and other finance related tasks.

Summary

IMEs are of significant use in the medicolegal arena. The multiple perspectives at play in an injury claim case contribute to a fair outcome. States have created successful insurance systems, and independent medical physicians play one of the many necessary roles. Should physicians enter the IME industry? Certainly they have the medical expertise and credentials to do so. The answer depends most heavily on the physician's ability to understand and adjust the attitudes and methods of his or her own clinical practice as those would mesh with the overall operation of an IME company.

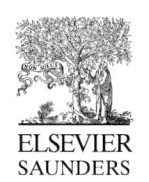

Legal Issues Affecting Ancillaries and Orthopedic Practice

David M. Glaser, JD

Fredrikson & Byron, P.A., 200 South Sixth Street #4000, Minneapolis, MN 55402, USA

Both the federal and state governments have imposed significant regulation on health care generally and on ancillary services in particular. This article focuses on how state and federal laws shape the ability of an orthopedic physician to offer ancillary services, whether as an individual, through a group practice, or as part of a joint venture. It focuses on how the Stark law, the Medicare anti-kickback statute, state anti-kickback, fee-splitting provisions, certificate of need laws, and various Medicare billing and supervision requirements impact the provision of ancillary services. It also briefly discusses how physicians should prepare for and respond to government investigations.

One factor that makes understanding the regulation so difficult is that the rules often define well-understood words in a counterintuitive way. For example, the word "referral" seems straightforward. According to the Stark law definition of "referral," however, a physician is deemed to have "referred" a patient to whoever provides the patient with a service ordered in the physician's plan of care. As a result, if one orders a film but does not offer any suggestion as to where the patient should receive the image, one is still considered to have "referred" the patient to the scanning facility the patient chooses.

Because of this complexity, and because the rules change so frequently, no one should rely on this article as the sole source of information about ancillaries. Analysis of each ancillary depends on its unique factors and also on state law. Therefore, it is impossible to present the issues in a format that is both comprehensive and easily comprehensible. One should consult with legal counsel rather than relying solely on the information presented here. This article, however, provides some basic information that may assist in the selection of counsel and in discussing options.

Tips for evaluating the quality of advice: separating myth from reality

Before discussing the specific laws, it is helpful to consider how a physician may determine whether a particular proposal is likely to be in compliance with the various laws. First, it is important for physicians to be cynical consumers of advice. There are a number of widespread myths about Medicare rules. When seeking advice from anyone, including attorneys, consultants, trade associations, or the government, it is important to recognize that many so-called "experts" often are incorrect. Just because conventional wisdom suggests something is right or wrong does not make it so. When seeking advice about any regulatory situation, one should ask for a citation to the underlying rule. The expert should be able to provide the applicable rule or, at a minimum, clearly articulate the rationale underlying his or her position.

Even a published rule is not necessarily valid. For Medicare, there is a very clear hierarchy of authority. The Medicare statute controls everything in the program, and the regulations interpret the statute. In addition to the statute and regulations, the Centers for Medicare and Medicaid Services (CMS, formerly the Health Care Financing Administration) publishes manuals such as the *Medicare Claims Processing Manual* and the *Medicare Beneficiary Manual* to help carriers and intermediaries interpret the law (These manuals

E-mail address: dglaser@fredlaw.com

replace the *Medicare Carriers Manual*.) Carriers and intermediaries, which are independent companies paid by the government to make most coverage decisions, are to use the instructions in these manuals to develop their policies. Carriers administer the Part B portion of Medicare, including physician services. Even though the manuals can be a useful tool for understanding Medicare's interpretation of the law, the statements in the manuals are not law; they are guidance. Finally, individual Medicare carriers issue publications that contain local policies. When something in a rule or policy contradicts something with greater legal authority, such as the Medicare statute, however, the rule or policy is invalid. Thus, although intermediaries and carriers have authority to create some policies, their authority is limited.

In fact, contractors frequently publish policies that exceed their authority. For example, nearly every Medicare carrier claims that "if it isn't written, it wasn't done." They use this statement to deny claims where documentation fails to meet the evaluation and management guidelines. Nothing in the law that supports this conclusion, however. In fact, this conventional wisdom is incorrect: nothing in the Medicare statute, regulation, or policy suggests that documentation is required for most Medicare services to be payable. (There are exceptions, however. Medicare rules do require documentation of the role of a teaching physician billing for services while supervising a resident.) In general, a lack of documentation alone should not permit a carrier to recover an overpayment or the government to recoup penalties for a false claim if the service actually was provided. In short, if a carrier takes a position that is unreasonable, one can and should challenge it. The Medicare appeals process is easy to use. If one works with experienced legal counsel, the appeal should more than pay for itself. (New rules governing Medicare appeals limit a physician's ability to introduce evidence that was not offered at the early levels of appeal. Therefore, in any appeal it is advisable to work with legal counsel before beginning the appeals process to ensure that all arguments are presented.)

In addition, whenever seeking advice, one should be careful to provide as much detail as possible about the facts, even details that seem irrelevant. Because of the unusual twists in the rules, information that may seem immaterial may affect the analysis dramatically. Imagine a scenario in which an orthopedic group is considering an MRI joint venture with a number of other physician groups. The group asks its legal counsel whether it is possible for several physician groups jointly to place an MRI in an offsite ambulatory surgical center (ASC). The answer: it would not be possible to image Medicare and Medicaid patients on a scanner located offsite in an ASC in an urban area. Over the course of discussion, however, it becomes clear that what the group referred to as an "ASC" was really a specialty hospital, jointly owned by the physicians and a local hospital. This fact completely changes the legal analysis of the proposed venture. What had first seemed to be impossible is, in fact, readily achievable. Even though common sense would never suggest that the facility's status as a specialty hospital, rather than an ambulatory surgical center, would impact the Stark analysis, this fact was definitive.

This story teaches two lessons. First, when seeking advice, it is essential to disclose all the relevant facts. There is a certain irony here: to know the relevant facts one must know all of the relevant law. Of course, if one knew all the relevant law, it would be unnecessary to seek advice. The best alternative is to disclose all conceivable facts and allow the expert to separate relevant facts from extraneous material. Second, because it will be necessary to disclose so much detail, it always is advisable to seek advice from an individual whom one can trust to have one's best interests at heart, such as one's lawyer or a well-respected and trustworthy consultant, rather than the Medicare carrier or another organization that may use the information against the health care provider.

There is one additional reason to be cautious when seeking regulatory advice from carriers: they are routinely inaccurate. Government studies have found that up to two thirds of inquiries receive incomplete or inaccurate answers. In one particularly egregious example, an investigator posing as a patient called to ask about coverage for a power wheelchair. Such chairs are covered if the patient "lacks sufficient trunk strength" to operate a manual chair. The caller asked the Medicare representative to explain what "trunk strength" meant. The answer: it relates to the size of the patient's car. The lesson: even "official" sources of information may not be accurate.

This section explored how to seek guidance. The next sections address the substantive law.

The Medicare anti-kickback statute

The Medicare anti-kickback statute makes it illegal for anyone to offer, solicit, make, or receive any payment that is intended to influence referrals under a federal health care program. Whenever an orthopod enters a venture with physicians or facilities that refer to or receive referrals from the orthopedic surgeon, it is necessary to consider the anti-kickback provisions. For example, suppose a radiology group proposed forming a limited liability company that would permit an orthopod to share in the profit on scans ordered by the orthopod. An anti-kickback analysis would be essential to this situation. The anti-kickback law is designed in large part to prevent someone (in this case the radiologist) from offering a financial incentive to use him or her for a service, rather than using a competing provider. The statute also would apply if a hospital offered an investment opportunity or a discount to a physician to encourage the physician to perform services at that facility. Nearly any relationship with a hospital, including medical directorships, leases, joint ventures, and consulting relationships, can trigger the statute. Even though these relationships can be perfectly legal, it is important to review them carefully.

Violating the anti-kickback statute is a felony, punishable by imprisonment, fines, and exclusion from the Medicare program. Because it is a criminal law, the key question in any anti-kickback case is the intent of the parties. The government must prove that the payment was intended to influence referrals. If the party making (or receiving) the payment did so with the belief it would influence referrals, the person has violated the law. When applying the law, the government uses the "one purpose" test. If there are several legitimate reasons for a payment, but one purpose of the payment is to influence referrals, the payment violates the statute.

The Medicare anti-kickback statute does not apply to payments made within a corporation. Therefore, the Medicare anti-kickback statute has no impact on how a practice divides revenue from ancillary services such as radiology, physical therapy, or an ASC that is owned entirely by the group practice. If, however, the ancillary services are being provided by a joint venture or similar arrangement in which payments are made from one corporation to another or from one individual to another, the anti-kickback statute can apply.

Because the government realizes that nearly every business relationship in the health care industry has the potential to violate the statute, it has published a number of safe harbors. The safe harbors are designed to protect arrangements in which the government feels that the risk of abuse is so low that it will not prosecute the venture, regardless of the intent of the parties. There are safe harbors protecting leases, ASCs, ventures in rural areas, personal service arrangements, and a number of other relationships. Each safe harbor has a number of elements.

To be protected by a safe harbor, one must satisfy completely each of its elements. Unfortunately, because the safe harbors are drawn quite narrowly, it is extremely rare for a venture to qualify for a safe harbor. For example, the safe harbor governing ASCs between a clinic and a hospital requires that the hospital "not be in a position to make or influence referrals directly or indirectly to any investor." CMS spokespeople have indicated that they believe a hospital has the ability to influence referrals inside the hospital's service area, so that this safe harbor would protect only an ASC joint venture placed outside the area. Because it is extremely unlikely that a hospital would place an ASC outside its service area, this safe harbor offers little practical protection.

There is a simple reason that the CMS has kept the safe harbors extraordinarily narrow. A relationship that meets a safe harbor is legal even if the parties' intent is to violate the statute. Because the government wants the ability to consider intent, it wants few relationships to qualify for safe harbor protection.

Although the conditions of a safe harbor often are difficult to meet, ventures that do not qualify for a safe harbor can still be perfectly legal. Each arrangement must be analyzed on a case-by-case basis to determine whether there is an improper intent to influence referrals. The analysis focuses purely on the parties' intent. Although it certainly is helpful to be close to satisfying the conditions of a safe harbor, relationships that are well outside of a safe harbor may be legal, and relationships that are almost within a safe harbor may be illegal.

As part of the Health Insurance Portability and Accountability Act, Congress required the Office of Inspector General (OIG) to issue advisory opinions about the anti-kickback statute. Unfortunately, there are some significant limitations on the advisory opinion process. First, the parties to the proposal must represent to the government that they intend to enter into the arrangement if the opinion is favorable. Second, the request must disclose all the relevant parties and facts. Third, the parties must agree to pay the government's fees. Fourth, and perhaps most importantly, the law prohibits the OIG from offering an opinion on whether the proposed payments are consistent with fair market value. Instead, the OIG simply issues its opinion based on the assumption that the payments reflect fair market value. The OIG is free, however, subsequently to challenge whether the payment is at fair market value. Because the single most important question in most transactions is whether the payments are at fair market value, there is a significant gap in the protection otherwise offered by the opinion.

It typically is possible to make a relatively reliable anti-kickback analysis without obtaining an advisory opinion. This possibility arises in part from one benefit of the advisory opinion program: it provides considerable insight into the OIG's view of certain transactions. Although the law makes it clear that only the parties who specifically requested the advisory opinion may rely on it, the existence of a favorable or unfavorable opinion allows counsel to assess better the risk associated with a particular structure. For example, the OIG has reviewed several proposed ASCs. The advisory opinions make it clear that even certain ASCs that do not qualify for safe harbor protection are unlikely to face challenge. The key issue is whether the structure of the ASC creates significant risk of overutilization of services. As long as that risk is low, the venture is unlikely to be contested.

Because the anti-kickback analysis is so fact driven, every fact is material. Transactions that seem justifiable may become very problematic as the result of one e-mail or conversation. For example, a device company may invite a physician to serve as a consultant. As long as the payment is consistent with the value of the physician's expertise, without taking into account the physician's status as a referring physician, this arrangement should not present a problem (unless a state law applies.) If the device company, however, were to say "because you are such a good customer, we want to reward you by having you serve as a consultant," an otherwise permissible relationship is suddenly highly questionable. The statement that the job is to "thank you" may suggest that the payments are, in part, related to referrals.

The bottom line is that there is seldom certainty in an anti-kickback analysis. Transactions rarely are clearly permissible or categorically prohibited. Rather, the analysis is highly fact specific and hinges on the motives of the parties.

Although the analysis may seem complex and burdensome, the availability of guidance such as advisory opinions usually makes it possible to make a qualitative assessment of the risk without incurring significant legal expense.

The Stark law

The Stark law is another federal law that affects the ability to provide ancillary services. The Stark law prohibits a physician from making any referral to an entity for the furnishing of a designated health service (DHS) if the physician or a member of the physician's immediate family has any financial relationship with the entity, unless the financial relationship fits within one of the law's exceptions. Stark also prohibits an entity from billing for any DHS furnished under a prohibited referral. Violations of the Stark law can result in penalties of up to $15,000 per claim.

Although that fine applies only to whoever submits a bill to the government, other penalties can apply to the physician who ordered the service. First, a scheme to circumvent the law can result in a $100,000 fine. In addition, the government could argue that various conspiracy provisions allow it to impose penalties on a physician who makes a prohibited referral, even if the physician is not billing for the service.

When it was passed, the Stark law was intended to be much clearer than the Medicare anti-kickback law. Unlike the anti-kickback law, the intent of the parties is irrelevant to a Stark law analysis. By avoiding the issue of intent, the Stark law was supposed to be simple and analytical: if there is a financial relationship that is covered by the law, the recipient of any referrals is prohibited from billing the Medicare or Medicaid programs for services, unless the relationship meets a Stark law exception. In reality, however, the Stark law often is far from clear because ambiguities about issues such as whether a payment is really at fair market value create considerable room for interpretation.

Part of the reason that the Stark law is so difficult to interpret is that many of the words used in the law contain detailed and counterintuitive definitions. As discussed earlier, the Stark law defines the word "referral" quite broadly: if a physician creates a plan of care, the physician is deemed to have referred the patient to whoever provides services pursuant to the plan, even if the physician does not explicitly mention the particular provider. For example, if a physician indicates that a patient requires crutches but does not name a particular vendor, the physician is deemed to have "referred" the patient to the ultimate provider of the crutch.

Other definitions are equally surprising. The law contains an exception that protects many referrals within a "group practice." It may seem easy to assume that the term refers to any clinic. As described in detail later, however, the law defines the term narrowly, creating a number of traps for unwary physicians. For example, if 25% of the services provided by members of the group practice are billed by another organization, the clinic will not qualify as a group practice. Groups that permit hospitals or other physician groups to bill for their physician services too frequently lose their ability to be a "group practice" under the Stark law.

Although the Stark law is often mentioned in the same breath as the anti-kickback statute, there are some very significant differences between the two laws. The anti-kickback statute is a criminal law, whereas the Stark law is civil; a Stark law violation results in monetary penalties, not imprisonment. (Unfortunately, the penalty of $15,000 per claim may feel like a criminal violation!) Second, unlike the anti-kickback statute, the Stark law applies even to payments within a physician's professional corporation. In short, the Stark law affects which ancillary services a clinic can provide and how it may divide clinic revenue.

The Stark law applies only to entities that provide DHS:

- Clinical laboratory
- Physical therapy
- Occupational therapy
- Radiology services
- Radiation therapy services and supplies
- Durable medical equipment and supplies
- Parenteral and enteral nutrition
- Prosthetics and orthotics
- Home health services
- Outpatient prescription drugs
- Inpatient and outpatient hospital services

Any organization that provides one of the listed DHS must determine whether it has any type of financial relationship with physicians who refer patients for the DHS. If it does, the relationship must fit within one of the Stark law exceptions. Alternatively, the entity must either stop billing Medicare and Medicaid for any services provided pursuant to a plan of care created by the physician or end the financial relationship with the physician.

The Stark law divides financial relationships into two categories: ownership and compensation. Some of the Stark law exceptions protect both types of financial relationships. Other exceptions protect only ownership and investment interests, whereas the remaining exceptions apply only to compensation arrangements. The next few sections elaborate on the Stark law exceptions.

Services provided within the clinic

For physician practices, the most important Stark law exception covers "in-office ancillary services." This exception covers both ownership and compensation relationships. If a physician group meets the exception's conditions, the physician practice can provide nearly all DHS. Under this exception a clinic may have an in-office radiograph or laboratory and provide physical therapy services to clinic patients.

Although the in-office ancillary exception is useful for most DHS, it cannot be used for most durable medical equipment (DME) or any parenteral and enteral nutrition. The only DME that can be provided under this exception are canes, crutches, walkers, and folding manual wheelchairs. In an urban area (which the Stark law defines as a county that is part of a metropolitan statistical area [MSA]; for a complete listing of MSAs, see http://www.census.gov/population/estimates/metro-city/acencty.txt), the only DME that a physician can sell to Medicare and Medicaid recipients are crutches, canes, walkers, and wheelchairs. Although the physician may dispense other DME to Medicare/Medicaid recipients, the physician cannot have any ownership interest in the DME company. (One also should be careful to avoid arrangements in which a DME supplier rents a closet or shelf from the physician. The OIG has indicated that these arrangements are inherently suspect.)

The Stark law definition of DME again illustrates that common sense can be misleading when dealing with Medicare. One might assume that all supplies paid for by the Durable Medical Equipment Regional Carrier are considered DME. In fact, however, prosthetics or orthotics are not considered DME. Therefore, if the clinic is considered a group practice under the Stark law, it can own and dispense braces and similar equipment to Medicare and Medicaid patients without running afoul of the law.

What is a "group practice?"

To qualify for the in-office exception, a number of conditions must be met. First, the services must be furnished personally by (or under the supervision of) a physician who is a member of the group practice. For these purposes, a group practice's physicians include employees and owners of the clinic and independent contractors.

Second, there are limits on where the services may be provided. By far the simplest test is that if all of the DHS provided at a location are billed by the clinic, then the location is considered a "centralized location" for the provision of DHS. If another organization bills for some of the DHS provided at that location, however, one of the tests below must be met.

If the clinic operates at least 35 hours each week and sees patients at least 30 hours a week in the same building as the equipment/location in question, then it should be possible to provide the DHS. This provision allows two clinics in a building to share services. If the DHS is across the street or down the block, however, it generally is difficult for two or more clinics to share it unless the arrangement meets the exception discussed later.

If the clinic operates in the same building less than 35 hours each week, it still may be possible to provide the DHS, but the requirements are considerably more complicated. First, the group or physician must operate at least 8 hours a week in the building. If this condition is satisfied, there are two alternative ways in which a clinic may provide DHS. First, services may be provided if the referring physician practices in the building at least 1 day a week, and the building is the principal place where referred patients see the physician. Alternatively, DHS may be provided if the physician or group members see patients at least 1 day a week, and either the service is ordered during a patient visit or a physician is present during the services.

The third element of the in-office exception requires that the services be billed either by the physician who performs or supervises the test, by the physician's practice itself, or by some entity that is owned wholly by the physician group.

Fourth, to use the in-office ancillary exception, a group must qualify as a "group practice" under the Stark law. To be considered a group, 75% of all services furnished by members of the group must be billed by the group. For this test, only W-2 employees and owners of the clinic are considered "members of the group"; independent contractors are not included. In other words, if the group allows other groups to bill for services provided by the group's physicians, either because the physician is moonlighting or performing outreach services, one must be certain that in aggregate no more than 25% of the services provided by anyone who is a shareholder, partner, or W-2 employee of the group are billed by the other organizations. The 75% figure can be calculated on the basis of time, revenue, or any other reasonable method as long as the method is chosen in advance. In addition, services provided in a Health Professional Shortage Area may be excluded.

Further, at least 75% of the clinic's patient encounters must be done by individuals who are considered members of the group. Again, W-2 employees and shareholders/partners of the group are both considered "members of the group"; independent contractors are not members of the group. As a result, if independent contractors provide 25% or more of the services billed by a group, the group cannot use the in-office ancillary exception. Small groups that use independent contractors on a regular basis must be wary of this requirement.

When looking at the "group practice" definition, it is important to note that the Stark law uses two very similar but distinct phrases: "members of the group" and "in the group." This distinction is another example of how very specific definitions drive a Stark law analysis. Independent contractors are considered to be "in the group," but they are not considered "members of the group." From a practical perspective, this means that independent contractors are permitted to supervise the delivery of DHS, but the services they perform do not count toward the 75% "group practice" tests.

Exceptions for ownership interests

Three exceptions permit physicians to own an entity that provides DHS. These exceptions pertain to publicly traded securities and mutual funds, ownership in a hospital, and rural providers.

Publicly traded securities and mutual funds

A physician may own stock in large publicly traded companies, such as those listed on large national and regional stock exchanges, that have stockholder equity of more than $75 million.

Ownership in a hospital

If a physician owns part of a hospital, and the physician is authorized to perform services at the hospital, the physician's ownership of the hospital is permissible even if the hospital provides DHS. The ownership interest, however, must be in the whole hospital and not in a subdivision of the hospital. (The Medicare Prescription Drug Improvement and Modernization Act of 2003 significantly limited this hospital ownership exception if the hospital is a "specialty hospital." That provision now has expired, and, as of this writing, ownership of a specialty hospital may satisfy the exception. CMS, however, has established a policy of refusing to license so-called "specialty hospitals.")

Rural providers

A physician may own an entity that provides DHS if the entity is located outside an MSA and at least 75% of all services provided by the entity are to people who live outside an MSA.

Compensation formula issues

In addition to putting restrictions on ownership interests, the Stark law limits the factors that can be included in compensation formulas. The biggest restriction is that compensation cannot reflect the volume or value of any referral for a DHS. For example, a physician should not receive credit in the compensation formula for radiologic tests, laboratory tests, physical therapy, occupational therapy, or any other DHS ordered by the physician and paid for under the Medicare or Medicaid programs unless the service is provided personally by the physician or meets the requirements of the "incident to" billing rules. (The "incident to" rules require a clinic physician to order the service and oversee the course of treatment. Further, the physician receiving credit for the service must be present in the office suite when the service is provided. CMS takes the position that services, such as radiology, that have a specific benefit under the statute may not be provided "incident to.")

The Stark law does not prohibit including profit from DHS in the pool of money available to the physicians; it simply places restrictions on how the pool of money may be divided. Revenue from DHS may be divided a number of ways. For example, it would be permissible to divide MRI revenue on the basis of evaluation and management and/or surgical production, or on seniority, or to divide it equally. It also is permissible to allocate profits from DHS among certain subgroups of the physician group, as long as no subgroup has fewer than five physicians. For example, in a multispecialty practice, it would be permissible to allocate the physical therapy revenue equally among the eight different orthopedic physicians even if other physicians in the group did not share in the revenue.

The key factor in a compensation analysis is that it is improper to credit any physician for ordering a DHS.

Because the Stark law rules define DHS as services reimbursed by Medicare or Medicaid, it is permissible to credit a physician for radiology, physical therapy, and other services as long as the patient is not covered by Medicare or Medicaid. Obviously, if a group chooses to use this approach, the group must be careful to be certain that no Medicare or Medicaid services are included accidentally in the compensation formula, unless those services meet the "incident to" requirements.

The Stark law requires the establishment of the compensation formula before applicable funds are received. If the group meets this condition, it may change the compensation formula at any time, as long as any changes to the formula are made before payment is received. Retroactive changes to the compensation formula are not allowed.

Exceptions that cover compensation relationships

Although there may be limits on compensation arrangements, the Stark law includes a number of compensation exceptions. In the interest of brevity, only the most commonly used exceptions are discussed in detail here.

Fair market value exception

The Stark regulations created a new exception for relationships if there is a written agreement signed by the parties describing all of the covered services and specifying the covered time period. The Stark law permits agreements to include a termination provision as long as the parties do not change the terms of the agreement more frequently than once each year. The compensation must be set in advance, consistent with fair market value, and may not be determined in any manner that takes into account the volume or value of referrals or other business generated by the referring physician. The rules also contain the rather obvious requirements that the arrangement not violate the Medicare anti-kickback statute or violate other federal laws.

Leases

A lease of office space or equipment is generally permissible if (1) it is in writing, specifying the details of the lease and signed by the parties; (2) the space or equipment leased is under the exclusive control of the lessee during the period of the lease; (3) the space or equipment leased is being used for a legitimate commercial purpose; (4) the term of the lease is at least 1 year; and (5) the rental charges are set in advance, consistent with fair market value, and are not determined in a manner that takes into account the volume or value of business or referrals between the parties. For purposes of determining the fair market value, the government asks what an individual with no referral relationship would pay for similar space or equipment. For example, if a lease involves space, the question is whether an accountant or lawyer would pay a comparable rent. In other words, the agreement should be commercially reasonable even if there were no referral relationship between the parties.

Employment

Payments to an employee are permissible if the payments reflect fair market value for the services and are not determined in any manner that takes into account the volume or value of referrals. There is no requirement that the employment agreement be in writing.

Personal service arrangements

Relationships with independent contractors are permissible as long as (1) the agreement is in writing, detailing the specifics of the agreement and signed by the parties; (2) the arrangement is effective for at least 1 year; and (3) the compensation is set in advance, does not exceed fair market value, and does not take into account the volume or value of referrals or business generated between the parties.

Non-monetary compensation of up to $300

Compensation that is not cash or cash equivalent of up to $300 per year (adjusted for inflation); in 2007, the cap is permissible as long as the physician did not solicit the compensation and the compensation is not determined in a manner that takes into account the volume or value of referrals or other business. This exception permits small gifts and free medical services, provided they do not violate the anti-kickback statute or other laws.

Additional exceptions

There also are a number of other exceptions protecting

- Relationships with hospitals and a group practice that pre-date December 19, 1989
- Arrangements with hospitals unrelated to the provision of DHS
- Certain physician incentive plans
- Physician recruitment and retention
- Isolated transactions such as the sale of a practice
- Certain relationships with academic medical centers
- Certain benefits worth $25 or less per episode that are incidental to membership in a medical staff
- Certain risk-sharing arrangements
- Compliance training

State law issues

In addition to federal laws, a number of state laws may affect the operation of any ancillary arrangement. Many states, such as Florida, have adopted laws that extend provisions of the Stark law and/or the Medicare anti-kickback law to all patients.

Further, most states have fee-splitting provisions. These laws may limit the sharing of revenue and frequently require physicians to notify patients about the physician's financial interest in the ancillary. In addition, some states have more unusual provisions. For example, Wisconsin has a provision that limits who may bill for many diagnostic tests.

Many states also have certificate of need (CON) laws that require government approval to purchase certain equipment or open new facilities. If one lives in a state with a CON, it is worth considering challenging the law. CON statutes are relics of cost-based reimbursement. Historically, Medicare paid many services (particularly hospital services) on the basis of the cost of the service. This reimbursement program created an incentive to build facilities without regard to need, because even if the new service was not used, the organization would recoup a large portion of its cost. Now, however, very few services are reimbursed on the basis of cost. If a physician acquires new equipment and there is insufficient demand, the physician bears the cost. CONs are antithetical to the notion on which the entire American economic system is based: that competition improves quality and lowers prices. Thus, physicians confronted by a difficult CON law should consider challenging it in court or lobbying for its repeal.

Because of the various obstacles that could be encountered, it is essential to consider state law before undertaking any ancillary service.

Insurance contracts

It is increasingly common for private insurers to include provisions in their managed care contracts that permit the insurer to deny payment for services at a new location or on new equipment unless the insurer gives preauthorization. Many physicians have purchased new equipment or opened a new ASC only to learn that their largest payor is unwilling to reimburse them for its use. Careful review of contracts is critical to prevent this problem.

Analysis of particular ancillary opportunities

The previous discussion has provided a general background of applicable federal and state law. This section addresses issues relating to common ancillary arrangements and opportunities.

Ambulatory surgical centers within a group practice

There is nearly no risk under any referral regulation associated with operating an ASC within a group practice. First, the Medicare anti-kickback statute does not apply to any payments within a group practice. Second, because ambulatory surgical services are not considered to be DHS under the Stark law, the Stark law is inapplicable. Therefore, unless a state statute creates additional restrictions, it should be possible to divide compensation from the ASC in almost any manner. For example, it is generally permissible to allocate the facility fee on the basis of professional production at the ASC. Although in most states an ASC within the group raises few legal issues, some state laws may create obstacles for ASCs. For example, a state's CON law may create a practical challenge to the formation of the ASC. Some states with CON laws, however, will permit facilities to avoid the CON process if the ASC is small enough or is located in the clinic. Therefore, it is important to understand state CON and other relevant laws, as well as any exceptions to those laws.

Ambulatory surgical center joint ventures

An ASC involving physicians from different professional corporations is also possible, although there are more significant legal issues involved than when the physicians are all within the same corporation. As discussed earlier, the Stark law does not apply because ASCs are not a DHS. The anti-kickback statute does apply to these joint ventures, however.

Because the Medicare safe harbors governing ambulatory surgical centers are extremely narrow, they seldom are of much assistance. In fact, the ASC safe harbors contain some unusual contradictions. One element of the safe harbor states that the opportunity to invest in the ASC should not be based on the investor's ability to refer. Another element of the safe harbor indicates that investors must perform services at the facility. It is extremely difficult to reconcile these two provisions. The first element suggests that if a physician ceases performing services at an ASC, it would be improper to end the physician's affiliation with the ASC. The second element would seem to require the ASC to terminate its relationship with the physician in this situation. CMS has not offered any insight into how to resolve this apparent contradiction. Given this lack of straightforward interpretation or guidance, legal counsel ultimately must use common sense to assess the risk associated with the structure of an ASC joint venture.

When structuring an ASC, there are a few pitfalls to avoid. First, do not "cherry pick" investors, punishing individuals who do not perform a sufficient number of cases at the facility. Be careful to avoid using pressure on an individual to change his or her referral patterns. In addition, be particularly careful in designing any marketing program for the ASC. As long as one exercises some care in structuring the ASC, it should be possible to form an ASC joint venture.

Referrals from unaffiliated physicians

There is a common misperception that it is illegal to accept referrals for DHS from physicians unaffiliated with the group. In most states, this notion is completely untrue: as long as the referring physician does not have any sort of financial relationship with the group, there is no legal barrier to the group's billing for scans, physical therapy, or other services performed at the request of another physician. Even if the referring physician does have some sort of financial relationship, such as a lease or independent contractor relationship with the group, one may accept referrals from the physician as long as the financial relationship qualifies for one of the Stark law exceptions. As with everything else, however, it is important to consider state law. Florida, for example, has a law that limits the number of outside referrals a physician can accept.

Radiology

Within the group

It is permissible for a medical group to own and operate radiologic equipment such as x-ray machines, MRIs, and other scanners.

The division of revenue from these tests, however, cannot be based on who ordered tests for Medicare or Medicaid patients. Instead, revenue should be divided evenly, based on E&M production, seniority, or any combination of these or other methods that is independent of who ordered the test.

If a clinic has exclusive control of the equipment at all times, the equipment can be placed at a remote location. If, however, any other entity is billing for some of the scans performed on the scanner, the location of the scanner becomes more important. It can be located in a building where the clinic operates at least 35 hours a week. If the clinic is open fewer hours at that location, there are significant restrictions on which patients may receive scans. These restrictions have been addressed previously in the discussion of the in-office ancillary exception.

For example, it is permissible for a clinic to operate an MRI at an off-site location, but only if all services provided at the MRI location are billed by the clinic. It is not permissible to bill Medicare or Medicaid for services provided at an off-site MRI shared with another clinic. (If state law permits it, an off-site joint venture MRI providing services to nongovernmental patients generally is permissible. If, however, any Medicare or Medicaid patients are referred between the parties, even if they are not included in the joint venture, it is important to analyze fully the Stark law and anti-kickback implications.)

If two clinics provide physician services in the same building, there is an argument they can share an MRI at that location and provide imaging to Medicare and Medicaid patients. Each clinic would bill for the scans it performs. Medicare allows such a venture as long as the clinic is supervising the scans for which it bills. These supervision rules are discussed in more detail later.

Radiology joint ventures

It is certainly possible to enter into radiology joint ventures. Ventures are easiest in rural areas. If the services are performed outside an MSA, and 75% of the patients live outside the MSA, joint ownership of the venture is possible. Even in cities, it is possible to enter into radiology joint ventures, but considerable care is necessary to make sure the arrangement is in compliance with both the Stark law and the anti-kickback law.

In November 2007, CMS issued new rules governing diagnostic tests. The new rules limit the ability of physicians to "mark up" certain diagnostic tests. In particular, physicians may not mark up any test performed "at a site other than the office of the billing physician." The new rules do not define the phrase "office of the billing physician" in any meaningful way. It appears that it may be possible for a physician to share and MRI in space leased part-time in a building where the physician has a clinic. However, because of the ambiguity in the rules, it is quite likely that Medicare will offer additional guidance on its interpretation of the regulation. The subsequent guidance may well impact the ability of physicians in separate clinics to share imaging equipment. Physicians considering or participating in a joint venture in an urban area will want to carefully monitor statements from CMS over the next few months.

Physical therapy and occupational therapy services

Because both physical therapy and occupational therapy are considered DHS under the Stark law, the division of revenue from these services may not be based on who ordered the service. One of the biggest misperceptions involving Medicare billing for therapy services is the belief that all physical therapy services must be billed "incident to" a physician's services. In fact, in the late 1990s, Medicare changed its rules to permit a physical therapist employed by a clinic to bill independently under the physical therapist's own name and billing number. Unfortunately, some Medicare carriers still insist that all physical therapy services provided by a clinic must be billed under the name and number of a supervising physician. Because the reimbursement is identical whether the services are billing under the name of the therapist or the physician, it might seem irrelevant which billing mechanism is used. In fact, there are significant advantages to billing under the name of the therapist.

To bill services as "incident to" a physician's services, several conditions must be met. First, one of the clinic's physicians must perform an initial service on behalf of the patient before any physical therapy service must be provided. This requirement makes it impossible for the therapist to see patients referred from other clinics unless one of the clinic's physicians first examines the patient.

Second, a physician from the clinic must be in the office suite at all times when therapy services are provided to Medicare patients. Finally, the "incident to" benefit cannot be used if services are provided in a hospital (including a hospital-based clinic) or skilled nursing facility. When services are billed under the name and number of the physical therapist, none of these three conditions applies.

There is only one benefit to billing physical therapy "incident to" a physician's service: "incident to" billing permits the supervising physician to receive credit for the physical therapy services.

Because there are compelling benefits to billing independently, any clinic providing physical therapy services to Medicare patients is well advised to consider billing the services under the name and number of the therapist, rather than the physician. Should the carrier claim it is not permissible for a physical therapist employed by a clinic to bill independently, work with legal counsel, contact the author, or contact CMS in Baltimore to obtain information to correct the carrier. This analysis focuses exclusively on Medicare rules. Because Medicaid rules vary from state to state, one must check the state's Medicaid rules relating to physical therapy services. One also should review private insurance contracts to determine whether they place any limits on such services.

Supervision and interpretation of and billing for diagnostic tests

Medicare (and, in many states, Medicaid) places a number of restrictions on the supervision of and billing for diagnostic tests. To bill Medicare for a diagnostic test, a physician or a member of the physician's group must personally perform or supervise the performance of the test.

Unless the physician or a member of the physician's group is supervising the test, any bill to Medicare must indicate that the test is a purchased diagnostic test. When a physician purchases a test, Medicare prohibits the physician from marking up the cost of the test on the Medicare claim; the physician must pass through the supplier's charge directly without any profit to the group.

Even though this rule applies only to Medicare claims, Medicaid programs in many states impose similar or even more restrictive rules. Finally, some private payors may have incorporated similar rules into their contracts.

In November 2007, Medicare issued new regulations that limit the ability of physicians to "mark up" either the professional or technical component of diagnostic tests in certain situations. A physician may not mark either the professional or technical component if it is performed in a location other than where the physician provides a full range of services. Medicare does not permit the physician to mark up the charge for the test. These rules were published recently and are poorly written. It is nearly impossible to determine how a clinic may charge for an MRI that is located in a freestanding building, in space controlled by the physician but used only for the MRI. (Once again, it is important to determine whether state Medicaid or any contracts with private insurers impose similar restrictions.)

Supervision of diagnostic tests

On April 19, 2001, Medicare issued a memorandum outlining the level of supervision required for every diagnostic test. The memorandum creates three different levels of supervision: personal, direct, and general.

For personal supervision a physician must be present in the room when the test is performed.

Direct supervision requires the presence of a physician somewhere in the office suite, although the physician need not be in the room where the test is performed. General supervision merely requires a physician to monitor the equipment periodically. The physician need not be present in the building when tests are performed.

The April 19 memorandum lists the level of supervision required for a wide range of diagnostic tests. If a test is not included in the memorandum, Medicare has indicated that only general supervision is required. Although many basic diagnostic tests such as radiographs and MRIs without contrast media only require general supervision, one should review the list to determine what level of supervision is required. For example, MRIs involving contrast require direct physician supervision.

Final thoughts on ancillary services and regulatory compliance

Operation of ancillary services is highly regulated. The rules and regulations are not always logical, but they are navigable. One should work with counsel who is familiar with the law. Be careful to disclose all relevant facts fully. Most importantly, ask questions: by being inquisitive one can determine whether the legal or consulting expert has a good understanding of the rules. If the physician and counsel work together, it usually is possible to structure the ancillary service in a way that can be both safe and profitable.

Preparing for and responding to investigations

Even if one takes great care to comply with laws and regulations, it still is possible that the government could question an ancillary service or other arrangement. Therefore, in addition to ensuring that one is in compliance with the law, it is crucial that staff and employees are prepared in the event of an investigation.

Although some investigations begin with an agent visiting the office or mailing a subpoena or other request for documents, in many cases the first contact with the government occur when an agent visits current or former employees of the clinic at the employee's home.

The agents prefer to conduct the visits at home for the same reason that a lion hunts at the rear of the pack: an employee at home is isolated and less able to seek help from friend. Because employees face the agents alone and with no advance warning, it is prudent to train all clinic employees on how to handle the visit. These visits put tremendous pressure on employees, who may worry (often needlessly) about their personal liability or about losing their job.

Although investigations often are completed with no penalty imposed, the mere investigation itself is a major burden. A staff member's panicked response to agents visiting his or her home can prolong an investigation, even if no laws have been violated.

It therefore is essential that everyone in the clinic be trained on how to handle contact from the government. Depending on the nature of the investigation, agents may contact administrators, medical professionals, billing staff, or receptionists. Because one cannot anticipate who will be contacted, one must make sure that absolutely everyone has received instructions on how to deal with investigators.

One may worry that raising the specter of a potential investigation will cause undue fear or suggest that the organization is doing something wrong. If the topic is discussed in a straightforward but light fashion, however, it can be an effective way to prepare employees in the event of an encounter with the government.

The training should cover the following tips:

- The basics of government investigations
- Recognizing the arguments that agents use to convince people to talk
- How an interview can go wrong
- The need for legal counsel
- An emergency response plan
- Informing the employer

The basics of government investigations

Inform the staff that although the odds of a government OIG visit are low, such visits are now becoming the norm in the health care industry. Emphasize that many of the investigations end without any penalties; the fact that the government is investigating does not mean that a violation has occurred.

Because the rules governing medical practices are complex and confusing, it is common for government agents and potential whistleblowers to misunderstand a rule. Therefore, they may believe a violation has occurred even when a practice is entirely legal. When an investigation starts, however, it is unclear whether the government is mistaken or whether there has in fact been a violation. Because of this uncertainty, it is important to prepare for the worst but hope for the best.

Recognizing the arguments that agents use to convince people to talk

Agents are very skilled at convincing people to submit to an interview. In some cases, the agents use fear to encourage cooperation. They might appeal to the employee's civic duty, arguing that the employee should help root out any wrongdoing. They might appeal to self-interest, arguing that unless the employee agrees to an interview, he or she will face prosecution. Agents typically will try to drive a wedge between the clinic and employees by telling employees that the clinic will try to blame them for the problem, so they might as well "save themselves" by turning on the clinic first.

In other situations, the agents will minimize the situation; for example, they may suggest that the visit is "just routine" and "not a big deal." This kind of statement is invariably at least a white lie: if the matter was not potentially significant, the agents would not be taking time out of their evening to conduct the visit. If staff members have been trained to anticipate the arguments the agents will use and understand why the agents are using them, it is less likely that the arguments will be effective. Inviting legal counsel to conduct some role-playing can help employees practice how to respond to potentially intimidating interview techniques.

How an interview can go wrong

Underscore the unwanted consequences of talking with an agent during an unexpected visit by talking about things that can go wrong in an interview with government agents.

First, even a small misstatement of the facts can cause major problems for both the employee and the practice, even if it is inadvertent. The error may cause the agent to doubt the credibility of every other statement, greatly prolonging the investigation. In some cases, the agent may accuse the person of making a false statement to the agent, which is a crime.

Second, miscommunication occurs frequently; that is, what the employee believes he or she said and what the agent heard are quite different. For example, in one investigation the employee was explaining how physician assistants saw the patient but the bill was submitted under the supervision physician's number. The witness thought nothing of it; it was typical "incident to" billing. The agent, however, interpreted this information as a suggestion that the physician was billing inappropriately for work she did not do.

Third, either the employee or the agent may have a poor understanding of the law. In one such situation, an agent mischaracterized the law, claiming that perfectly legal activities were illegal. The employee, naively trusting that a government agent's characterization of the law would be correct, concluded that he had violated the law. He then "confessed" to activities that were perfectly legal. The way the agent worded the confession made it sound as if the employee had broken the law knowingly. It can be very, very difficult to reverse the impact of this type of "confession," even if there has been no violation.

The need for legal counsel

For all of the reasons reviewed here, it is prudent for a staff member to seek legal advice before engaging in any interview with a government agent. Once approached by the government, the staff member should contact legal counsel immediately. Legal representation is crucial to an effective response to an investigation, and the staff member should refrain from answering any questions until legal counsel is present.

It also is important for employees to understand that unless the agent produces a search warrant, the government cannot make them do anything before they contact legal counsel. On most visits, agents will not have a subpoena or other written document; they simply will ask the employee to speak voluntarily. Even if the agent does have a document such as a civil investigative demand or a grand jury subpoena, that document does not require the employee to do anything before contacting legal counsel. In fact, although the OIG does have the right to "immediate access" to records, the law defines "immediate access" as 24 hours.

In the unlikely event that an agent has a search warrant, the agent is entitled to take documents. Otherwise, it is entirely permissible to send the agent away. Before doing so, however, one should be sure to get the agent's business card. One will want to know who is conducting the investigation.

An emergency response plan

If an employee is contacted, there is a very real possibility that other employees are being contacted at the same time. Make sure employees know whom to call if they are contacted and that they understand the importance of contacting that person immediately. Because there may be other visits set to occur at the same time, the call should be made within minutes, rather than hours. Then, make certain that your contact person has a plan for reaching legal counsel and other employees on very short notice.

Make sure employees have a number of contact options if one or more people are unavailable. Everyone should understand that a visit from an OIG agent merits an immediate response, even if polite (or shaken) employees are reluctant to bother a colleague at home.

Informing the employer

It is particularly important that staff members understand that it is permissible for them to tell the employer if they are contacted by an agent. Some agents will close an interview by asking the subject to keep the visit confidential. They may say something like, "It will make it more difficult for me to conduct my investigation if people learn of it," which implies it would be obstruction of justice to disclose the government contact. Disclosure of government contact is not obstruction of justice. Rather, it is perfectly legal for someone to reveal that he or she has been contacted by the government. If employees remain silent, physicians may not learn of the investigation for months. Thus, it is crucial that employees know that it is permissible and important for them to tell their employer if they have been contacted by the government.

Final thoughts on investigations

It is important to revisit this topic frequently. Many organizations train staff on how to handle contact with a government agent once but then do not repeat the training for years. In addition to the need to train new employees on these procedures, one should keep in mind that the pressure of an actual investigative visit makes it very hard for employees to follow the guidance, even when the training is fresh. If the training occurred many months before the OIG agent's visit, it is quite possible that employees will not recall all the points that were covered.

Many complex factors go into determining how best to respond to an investigation, including the nature of the investigation (civil or criminal), the relative culpability (or lack thereof) of the client, and the nature and quality of the evidence. The initial contact often is critical. When clients undertake the initial communications directly with the OIG—without adequate preparation or understanding of the legal issues—the results can be disastrous. An experienced advisor should guide the client through the process, including development of an appropriate communications strategy, analysis of the evidence, determination of how to structure relations with employees and other relevant parties in the investigation, and whether to pursue early negotiations or articulate grounds for the government to decline prosecution.

There is no way that a surprise government visit can be viewed as a good thing, but with careful preparation one can minimize its impact.

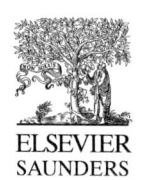

The Attack on Ancillary Service Providers at the Federal and State Level

Robert Cimasi, MHA, ASA, CBA, AVA, CM&AA, CMP

Health Capital Consultants, 9666 Olive Boulevard, Suite 375, St. Louis, MO 63132, USA

The health care delivery system in the United States perhaps has witnessed more dramatic changes during the last decade than it had since the passage of Medicare. Technological advances have made it possible for more procedures to be provided on an outpatient basis. The managed care revolution and changes in reimbursement for Medicare services have forced providers to look for more efficient ways to provide services as well as for additional sources of revenue- and margin-producing business. The move toward specialized inpatient and outpatient facilities, often owned by physicians, is a natural reaction to these significant changes. These technological advances, together with the cuts in reimbursement for professional services by managed care organizations and the Medicare Resource-Based Relative Value Scale, have resulted in increasing physician ownership of ancillary services and technical component revenue streams. These developments have resulted a "turf war" between physicians and hospitals over who should control these revenues. The government, as the largest health care payor in the United States, often views high-profit provider levels as inherently unreasonable. The development of specialty and niche providers, rather than posing a threat to the health care delivery system, is an innovation that allows health care services to be provided in a more cost-effective manner while maintaining and improving quality and beneficial outcomes and providing beneficial competition to established hospitals and other providers.

Much skepticism still remains in the health care industry about the benefits and role of market competition, however. In response to fears that unbridled competition may harm the health care system, the Federal Trade Commission (FTC) and the Department of Justice (DOJ) recently conducted extensive hearings on competition in health care. The agencies reminded state and local regulators and the health care industry that competition has affected health care quality and cost-effectiveness positively and recommended removing many of the barriers to competition that prevent it from fully benefiting consumers [1]. Despite the clear benefits of competition in health care, hospitals feel very threatened by specialty and niche providers. Their fear that these providers will "cherry-pick" and "cream-skim" the most profitable patients and procedures has caused hospitals to mount attacks against specialty and niche providers at the local, state, and federal levels.

The hospital industry also seems to be using its negotiating strength to induce insurance companies to exclude these providers. Additionally, the industry is using the media to stoke the public's fears of the closure of local hospitals. It often plays on the myth of greedy physicians ordering unnecessary procedures in contrast to benevolent community-oriented not-for-profit hospitals. In the wake of an epidemic of tens of thousands of deaths each year caused by medical errors [2], the general hospitals' unfounded charges that physicians would perform unnecessary procedures highlights the current state of the attack on specialty and niche providers, including surgical hospitals.

Government regulators' struggle to keep pace with the changes in the health care delivery system has led to an inconsistent regulatory scheme. Providers are subject to different regulations based on the state in which they are located and also are subject to differing regulations based on

E-mail addresses: rcimasi@healthcapital.com; asharamitaro@healthcapital.com the type of services they provide. These differences have resulted in a schizophrenic regulatory framework. Coupled with the inconsistent manner in which Medicare reimburses providers, this situation illustrates the law of unintended consequences; that is, when governments try to solve one problem, they often end up causing others. Because regulations are not developed in a coordinated manner, different levels of government often end up working against each other's interest. The potential conflict between certificate of need (CON) and antitrust laws is a prime example of this problem.

Ownership provides physicians with the opportunity to have more control over their professional work environment, work schedule, and clinical practice. In the recent American Hospital Association (AHA) case study of the Oklahoma City health care market, an unnamed physician-investor of a niche facility is quoted as saying, "I love being able to control my schedule. Between surgeries, I can have a cup of coffee, dictate notes and call my office; and when I walk in to see the second patient, everything is ready to go" [3]. This second-guessing of physicians' motivations illustrates the profound anti-physician attitudes of many hospital executives.

Physicians are motivated to invest in specialty and surgical hospitals not only to obtain better lifestyles; they also are reacting to reductions in the reimbursement for physician services. During the 1990s, although most professions saw an increase in their compensation, physician compensation was stagnant. Most of the propaganda from the hospital industry about specialty and niche providers plays on the public's fears of greedy physicians. Physician investors in specialty and niche providers often are seeking to replace reductions in reimbursement resulting from managed care or from the changes in Medicare payment levels for professional services. The assumption underlying much of the fear of specialty and niche providers is that physicians who invest their own money in health care and seek to earn a profit are bad, an odd assumption in a capitalist society.

These issues frame the battle between physicians and hospitals over who should get to control and profit from technical component revenue streams. At its heart, the controversy over specialty and surgical hospitals is a turf war between physicians and hospitals over the technical component revenues from procedures and diagnostic testing.

Discernable trends and overview of recent developments

The turf war between hospitals and physicians is the catalyst driving the increasingly volatile regulatory environment surrounding niche providers. In attempting to protect what they perceive as their "turf," hospitals have united in their battle against specialty and niche providers. Both the AHA, representing not-for-profit hospitals, and the Federation of American Hospitals, representing investor-owned for-profit hospitals, are waging national and local public relations campaigns against what they term "limited services providers." In contrast, physician organizations are split on this issue because of interspecialty conflicts and the distraction of the medical malpractice crisis. This lack of agreement and focus has prevented the formation of a unified front against hospitals' attempts to monopolize technical component revenues.

Hospitals' attack on specialty and niche providers manifests itself in a number of different ways at both the state and federal levels of government. The primary means of attack has been by limiting the exceptions to the Stark law and the anti-kickback statute. As discussed later in this article, Congress has specifically exempted certain financial arrangements from Medicare fraud and abuse laws to protect arrangements that have positive effects and pose little or no risk of abuse. Opponents of specialty and niche providers urge the federal government to eliminate some of these exceptions, including the "whole hospital" exception.

Some of the changes in Medicare reimbursement for outpatient services may be characterized as attacks on specialty and niche providers. These may not be frontal attacks, but they are, in fact, attacks because their effect is felt primarily by freestanding facilities and not by hospital-based outpatient departments. Freestanding facilities are more often physician-owned specialty or niche providers. Therefore, changes in Medicare reimbursement for outpatient services represent a backdoor attack on these providers.

Medicare's fee schedule for ambulatory surgical centers (ASCs) is still based on 1986 cost surveys adjusted yearly for inflation, making it possible that payments are not consistent with costs [4]. A February 2003 report issued by the Health and Human Safety Inspector General urged the Centers for Medicare and Medicaid Services (CMS) to set consistent reimbursement levels for hospital outpatient departments (HOPD) and freestanding ASCs [5]. In two thirds of the procedures examined in the report, all of which can be performed in either setting, HOPDs were reimbursed more than ASCs for the same procedures. The median overpayment was $282. This discrepancy results in overpayments to hospitals of $1 billion dollars annually. Overpayments to ASCs for the remaining procedures accounted for $100 million annually. The AHA argued in response that hospitals need to be overpaid to support their emergency rooms, ICUs, 24-hour service, charity care, and generally sicker patients [5]. The merger payment levels for HOPDs and ASCs have not been included in the 2003 Medicare bills. Furthermore, the Medicare Payment Advisory Commission (MedPAC) recommendation to cap outpatient surgery payments was not included in the 2003 Medicare Act [6].

One of the primary attacks on specialty and niche providers on a state level is through the use of CON laws. Because CON laws stifle competition and innovations in the delivery of health care services, it is not surprising that specialty and niche providers are more prevalent in states without CON regulations. A stringent CON regulation can effectively prevent or limit specialty and niche providers from entering a state, thereby protecting general hospitals from competition. A CON regulation often includes different review criteria for hospital providers than for physician organizations seeking to add new equipment or services.

CON regulations are not the only way the hospital industry is attacking specialty and niche providers on the state level. One of the most pernicious recent attacks is the New Jersey ASC tax enacted in 2004. Under this tax, physicians are subsidizing care provided in hospitals. When physicians provide charity care services in hospitals, the hospital often bills and is reimbursed for these same patients. It is interesting that the tax is applied only to ASCs, diagnostic imaging centers, and cancer treatment centers and does not apply to for-profit hospitals.

Justification for many of these attacks is being sought under the guise of promoting quality and charity care. The hospital industry currently is engaged in a large-scale public relations battle to shift the blame for medical errors and accusations of providing too little charity care away from hospitals. There has been increasing scrutiny of the levels of charity care provided in exchange for granting hospitals tax-exempt status. Additionally, in 22 states suits have been filed against tax-exempt hospitals, alleging they violate their tax-exempt status by charging uninsured patients higher rates than insured patients who have discounted fee-for-service contracts [7].

These charges come in the wake of an ongoing national controversy over several recent studies finding that medical errors are a leading cause of death. The Institute of Medicine's 1999 study reported that as many as 44,000 to 98,000 deaths may be linked directly to medical errors [8]. Indeed, deaths related to hospital infections are the fourth leading cause of mortality according to the United States Centers for Disease Control and Prevention. An investigation by the *Chicago Tribune* found that nearly three quarters of these hospital infections were preventable [9]. During the last several years, the Institute of Medicine report and others have increased public awareness of medical errors [10]. A recent study by the US Agency for Healthcare Research on 18 types of hospital complications "sometimes caused by medical errors" found that "postoperative infections, surgical wounds accidentally opening and other often-preventable complications lead to more than 32,000 U.S. hospital deaths and more than $9 billion in extra costs annually" [11].

In light of these recognized hospital problems with quality and charity care, the current attack on limited-service providers including surgical hospitals and diagnostic imaging centers (both of which have a well-documented history of quality improvements and cost savings) is disingenuous at best.

Impact of the specialty hospital moratorium and its June 2005 expiration

Recent years have seen increases in the numbers of specialty and niche providers. In an April 2003 report, the Government Accountability Office (GAO) identified 92 existing cardiac, orthopedic, surgical, and women's specialty hospitals in operation as of February 2003 [12]. GAO researchers additionally noted that the number of specialty hospitals has tripled since 1990, with at least another 20 specialty hospitals under development [12]. Although specialty and niche providers are not a new phenomenon, the increase in their numbers has led to concerns in the hospital industry that they will cream-skim or cherry-pick the most profitable patients and procedures away from community hospitals. At the FTC/DOJ Hearings on Health Care and Competition Law and Policy, former CMS administrator Thomas Scully stated, "…when I drive around the country and see where

ASCs are popping up, I can tell you who we're overpaying" [13]. Although health care traditionally has been regulated by the states, the federal government, as the largest payor of health care services, can mandate how health care services are provided in the United States.

This fear on the part of the part of hospitals seems to have led to the mounting of numerous attacks on specialty and niche providers in Congress and state legislatures. At the heart of these battles is the technical component of diagnostic services and procedures. Some attacks, such as the "designated imager" proposals, are part of a turf war between radiologists and other specialists over technical component revenues. Other attacks, such as the specialty hospital moratorium, are part of the war between full-service community hospitals and specialty hospitals over those coveted, "profitable" Medicare patients.

The specialty hospital moratorium contained in the Medicare Prescription Drug, Modernization, and Improvement Act of 2003 (MMA) is the most significant attack on physician-owned facilities since the enactment of the Stark laws. The moratorium applies only to specialty hospitals, but the justification for the moratorium, protecting community hospitals from cream-skimming, could just as easily apply to other physician-owned specialty and niche providers such as ASCs and diagnostic imaging centers.

The MMA's 18-month moratorium on the development of new specialty hospitals was the culmination of several years' battle against the so-called "loop-hole" in the Stark laws allowing physicians to have ownership interests in hospitals (ie, the whole-hospital exception) [14]. The temporary moratorium seemed to represent a compromise between the faction wanting to eliminate the whole-hospital exception for all hospitals and the faction concerned only with the perceived threat from specialty and niche providers.

In April 2003, the GAO issued its first report on the market share and physician ownership of specialty hospitals. The GAO found that specialty hospitals represented a growing share of the hospital market and that the number of specialty hospitals has grown rapidly [15]. The GAO also found that 70% of all specialty hospitals were owned by physicians. The GAO issued a more detailed report in October 2003 analyzing the impact of specialty hospitals on general hospitals.

In implementing the moratorium the GAO confirmed that of the specialty hospitals that did not apply for a grandfather determination, only six physician-owned specialty hospitals were under development, although the AHA and Federation of American Hospitals had tentatively identified 52 facilities as potential physician-owned specialty hospitals under development [16]. Five of these six specialty facilities were scheduled to be surgical hospitals; one was scheduled to be a cardiac hospital. All six of the specialty hospitals are located within three states: two in California, one in South Carolina, and three in Texas. Because there was insufficient information to determine the status of 17 of the potential 52 facilities, there could be as many as 23 specialty hospitals under development that have not applied to the CMS for grandfather determination. Of the 40 applications from specialty hospitals under development and seeking grandfather determination under the MMA moratorium, the CMS approved 12 of the facilities; 25 of the applications are pending.

The 18-month specialty hospital moratorium that began on December 8, 2003 [17] ended officially on June 8, 2005 [18]. The expiration of this ban did not go unnoticed, however, and there is still strong contention on both sides of the debate [17]. Additionally, the expiration of the moratorium continues to promulgate an uncertain regulatory environment for joint ventures involving specialty and niche providers. The ever-changing regulatory environment and the resulting effects of competition among hospitals and physicians are highly debated among health care economists, provider groups, health administrators, and the media. For example, a *Modern Healthcare* article predicted that lifting the specialty hospital moratorium might result in a doubling of the currently existing 100 specialty hospitals [19]. Conversely, an environmental assessment by the American College of Physicians reports that "The national market share of specialty hospitals will not increase significantly in the short term despite the expiration of the moratorium on new physician-owned hospitals contained in the Medicare Modernization Act of 2003" [20]. Therefore, physicians considering joint ventures with niche providers must be aware of the uncertain regulatory environment affecting the specialty provider industry.

United States Senate bill to reinstate the moratorium

Complicating the already murky regulatory environment is a bill to reinstate the moratorium.

An original bill to provide for reconciliation pursuant to Section 202(a) of the concurrent resolution on the budget for fiscal year 2006 was passed on December 12, 2005, and includes a renewal of the moratorium until the earlier of (1) the date that the Secretary submits the final report under subsection (b)(2) or (2) the date that is 6 months after the date of the enactment of this Act [21].

Centers for Medicare and Medicaid Services' refusal to certify new specialty hospitals for Medicare reimbursement

Equally compounding the debate surrounding the state of the specialty hospital moratorium is the CMS refusal to certify new specialty hospitals for Medicare reimbursement [18]. The CMS is withholding the ability to receive Medicare payments from newly opened specialty hospitals, although the end of the moratorium lifted the prohibition on new market entry of physician-owned specialty hospitals. With powerful interests on both sides of this debate, it is uncertain what the future holds for specialty hospitals. This lack of clarity only compounds the already uncertain regulatory environment surrounding specialty facilities and is another factor that must be weighed in valuing these facilities. The CMS declared that it and its regional offices around the country will not issue payment agreements to any new specialty hospitals, so even were a facility to open, it would be unable to collect payments for treating Medicare and Medicaid patients. Effective June 9, 2005, the CMS informed the Medicare fiscal intermediaries not to process any new Medicare provider enrollment applications (CMS-855A forms) for specialty hospitals and not to forward recommendations for approval of CMS-855As for these hospitals to the CMS regional offices or State Survey Agencies. In addition, any new specialty hospital receiving accreditation as a hospital by the Joint Commission on Accreditation of Healthcare Organization or the American Osteopathic Association may not receive approval to participate in Medicare until a recommendation for approval of the CMS-855A is received in the regional office [22]. During this time the CMS will begin implementing the following changes: (1) reform payment rates for inpatient hospital services through Diagnosis Related Group (DRG) refinements and ASCs; (2) more closely scrutinize whether entities meet the definition of a hospital; and (3) review procedures for approval for participation in Medicare [23].

United States Congressional initiatives

On October 7, 2005, US Representative Wally Herger (R-CA) introduced the "Ambulatory Surgical Center Payment Modernization Act of 2005," (HR 4202) in the US House of Representatives, with identical legislation being proposed by Senator Crapo (R-ID) in the Senate (S 1884) [24]. The proposed legislation would replace the current list of procedures authorized to be provided in ASCs with a much narrower list of procedures that cannot be performed by ASCs. Additionally, the legislation would connect ASC payment rates to 75% of the rates paid to hospital outpatient departments for identical services, with specific phases for incorporating the special payment rules over 4 years to avoid disruptive cuts in payments and industry stability [25].

Earlier, on August 9, 2005, Senators Charles Grassley (R-IA) and Max Baucus had sent a letter to their Senate colleagues contending that, "When physicians are able to refer patients to health care facilities they own, a potential conflict of interest is created between the clinical needs of the patient and the financial interests of the physician-owner" [26]. The Senators added that the "Hospital Fair Competition Act of 2005" (S 1002) introduced in May "would level the playing field to allow for true competition" in health care [26]. Specifically, the bill introduced in May 2005 would prohibit physician-owners from referring Medicare and Medicaid patients to new specialty hospitals [27] and would be retroactive to June 7, affecting any specialty hospital built between then and the bill's passage [18]. The bill additionally ordered re-examination or recalculation of DRGs, one of the main reasons opponents to physician-owned specialty hospitals believe health care providers prefer to offer some services rather than others [28].

Another congressional initiative took place during the summer of 2005. On July 28, 2005, three leading House Democrats sent a letter to CMS Administrator Mark McClellan asking the CMS to review specialty hospitals for racial bias and to continue the moratorium on certifying new physician-owned specialty hospitals [29]. The letter cites a study purporting to show that, in 2000, 3.6% of Medicare patients in physician-owned cardiac hospitals were African American, as compared with 9.6% of Medicare patients at general acute-care hospitals.

Medicare Payment Advisory Commission recommends extending the moratorium until 2007

MedPAC published a full report in March 2005 examining the costs and use of physician owned specialty hospitals. The March 2005 report made the following recommendations, including

(1) The Secretary should improve payment accuracy in the hospital inpatient prospective payment system by: (a) Refining the current DRG's to more fully capture differences in severity of illness among patients, (b) Basing the DRG relative weights on the estimated cost of providing care rather than on charges, and (c) Basing the weights on the national average of hospitals; relative weights on the estimated cost of providing care rather than on charges, and (d) Basing the weights on the national average of hospitals' relative values in each DRG.
(2) The Congress should amend the law to give the Secretary authority to adjust the DRG relative weights to account for differences in the prevalence of high-cost outlier cases.
(3) The Congress and the Secretary should implement the case-mix measurement and outlier policies over a transition period.
(4) The Congress should extend the current moratorium on specialty hospitals until January 1, 2007.
(5) The Congress should grant the Secretary the authority to allow gainsharing arrangements between physicians and hospitals and to regulate those arrangements to protect the quality of care and minimize financial incentives that could affect physician referrals [30].

In addition to recommendations in the MedPAC 2005 report to extend the moratorium for further study and to rebalance DRG payment levels, the report made several significant findings:

1. Physician control was a primary motivator for physician ownership of specialty hospitals, because they believed greater control would elicit greater productivity and efficacy, including fewer disruptions to the operating room schedule; less down time between surgeries; heightened ability to work between two operating rooms during a block of operating room time; and more direct control of the operating room and staff.
2. "Physician-owned heart, orthopedic, and some surgical hospitals tended to treat fewer Medicaid patients than peer hospitals and community hospitals in the same market. Heart hospitals treated primarily Medicare patients, while orthopedic and surgical hospitals treated primarily privately insured patients".

Medical community attacks: designated imaging regulations, economic decredentialing of niche provider and facility requirements

The issue of in-office ancillary imaging pits radiologists against other physicians. Increasingly radiologists face increased competition from referring physicians [31]. A study funded by the Radiological Society of North America and presented in 2004 claimed that self-referral leads to increased use of diagnostic imaging. The study recommended that the radiologist professional community lobby the federal government to enact regulations making self-referrals more difficult. According to the chief researcher, David C. Levin, "Orthopedic surgeons really don't belong in the business of owning MR scanners" [32].

The American College of Radiology (ACR) recently announced plans to lobby for legislation requiring Medicare to define standards for physicians performing diagnostic imaging [33]. At a December 2004 meeting, MedPAC staff members stated, "It's important for CMS to set national standards for each imaging modality" [34]. MedPAC endorsed relying upon private accreditation agencies to develop the standards [34]. Private accreditation agencies would most likely be organizations such as the ACR, which currently accredits radiology departments. ACR facility accreditation for a specific imaging modality requires that physicians who interpret diagnostic imaging studies meet ACR qualifications for that modality [35].

Economic decredentialing is yet another tactic used by the medical community to attack physician owners of specialty hospitals. The landmark state and national health care debate involving New Albany Surgical Hospital in Ohio serves as a prototypical model for the kind of economic back-stabbing hospitals have engaged in against their medical staff physicians under the guise of "economic credentialing." In January 2004 OhioHealth, an eight-hospital health system, revoked the hospital privileges of 17 staff physicians who were investors in the competing for-profit specialty hospital [36].

It is well established that a hospital may exercise some degree of control over the identity and number of physicians to whom it grants staff privileges (ie, granting and revoking staff privileges based on physician qualifications and quality of care controls) [37]. In a response to the growing prevalence of specialty hospitals such as ASCs, however, general hospitals are engaging in a new form of credentialing termed "economic credentialing." Although the term "economic credentialing" does include such economic factors as the frequency of physician's use of the hospital and the physician's ability to use hospitals facilities in an economically efficient manner, it recently has begun to include such retaliatory practices as the removal from the hospital medical staff of doctors who have a financial interest at a competing specialty facility. Hospitals that do not go as far as blatantly revoking the staff privileges of physicians who have a financial interest in a nearby specialty hospital nevertheless participate in the attack on specialty hospitals by refusing to grant the specialty hospital the needed transfer agreement, thereby engaging in another form of economic credentialing.

It is precisely this economic testing of physician hospital staff privileges, without regard to quality of care, and the refusal of needed transfer agreements to nearby specialty hospitals that allow general hospitals to prevent specialty hospitals and niche providers from entering the health care marketplace. Because physicians have been generally unsuccessful in safeguarding against the encroachment of economic factors into the credentialing process, the number of similar cases upholding the hospitals' discretionary economic practices has been growing rapidly. For example, in *Lister v Methodist Medical Center*, the court upheld a hospital's closed-staff policy for anesthesia services, stating, "The by-laws do not limit the hospital from taking actions which affect the plaintiff's staff privileges unrelated to the competency or conduct. The parties concede that the hospital decided to terminate plaintiff's clinical privileges solely due to business considerations, an entitled deference" [38]. Both parties "stipulated that the decision to preclude the plaintiff from exercising his clinical privileges [was] unrelated to any question of confidence of quality of anesthesia services provided" [38].

Hospitals' use of economic credentialing has severe and wide-ranging effects on both quality of care and freedom of competition in the health care marketplace. By trying to stifle the emergence of more-efficient specialty hospitals, hospitals are in effect using their established but inefficient system to stifle innovative health care delivery models [39].

Other state-level attacks on ambulatory surgery centers

In June 2004, the New Jersey legislature imposed a tax on certain ambulatory care facilities, specifically excluding those owned by a hospital. The measure imposed a 3.5% tax on gross revenues of ambulatory care centers and a 6% tax on gross receipts from cosmetic procedures. The revenues raised by the assessment will compensate hospitals for charity care. Facilities taxed include ASCs, facilities providing diagnostic imaging services, and outpatient cancer centers [40]. The Medical Society of New Jersey opposed the legislation vigorously because it imposed an additional level of taxation on the physician-owners of these facilities. The facility itself is taxed under the corporate business tax, and the physician-owners are taxed under the personal income tax code [41]. Physicians remain uncompensated for the charity care provided in a hospital [42].

In February 2005, a bill was introduced in the Missouri state senate which would modify provisions of the law applying to ASCs and would require that an ambulatory medical treatment center that performs surgical procedures, childbirth services, cardiac catheterizations, or endoscopy have a "working agreement" with a local hospital for emergency patients. The legislation was supported by the Missouri Hospital Association (MHA), which launched a grassroots advocacy program throughout Missouri addressing what it termed "limited service providers" by producing briefing papers for the Missouri legislature claiming that limited-service providers have little state supervision and that the physician-owners of these facilities have a financial incentive to cherry-pick patients [43].

Certificate of need

The Florida legislature passed a bill prohibiting the licensure of new specialty hospitals. A hospital may not be licensed if 65% of its patients received cardiac, orthopedic, or cancer services or if it restricts its medical and surgical services primarily to cardiac, orthopedic, surgical, or oncology specialties [44]. Although ASCs are not specifically covered by the moratorium, the moratorium is a significant victory for the hospital industry in its battle to protect hospitals from limited-service providers. It has "emboldened [hospital lobbyists] to the extent they're now linking ASCs with specialty hospitals in [certificate of need] fights," writes Lorin Patterson, a partner in the health care practice at Shook, Hardy, and Bacon in Kansas City, MO in a recent *HealthLeaders* article [45].

Public relations attacks against niche providers and organized medicine's fragmented response

Although the hospital industry is united in its public relations campaign against specialty hospitals, differences among the medical specialties have prevented physicians from mounting a unified front against the hospital industry. The American Medical Association's (AMA) September 10, 2004 "Presentation to the Council on Health Care Economics and Policy on Specialty Hospitals, Ambulatory Surgery Center, and General Hospitals: Charting Wise Public Policy," highlights the AMA's support of specialty hospitals [46]. The presentation emphasized that it supported a "level playing field" between general and specialty hospitals and that the completion between health care providers "promotes delivery of high-quality, cost effective health care" [46]. Additionally, the AMA highlighted its official AMA Ethical Opinion that physicians may refer patients to a facility if they directly provide care or services at the facility or if a demonstrated need exists in the community [46].

Intrinsic to its support of leveling the playing field, the AMA noted that the April 2003 the GAO concluded that half of the specialty hospitals with physician ownership were owned by individual physicians with a share of less than 2%. Moreover, the AMA underscored the fact that many general hospitals channel patients through integrated delivery systems and primary practices, as well as exclusive credentialing and medical staff development plans [46]. Finally, the AMA reiterated that it opposes efforts to stifle competition by terminating medical staff privileges because of direct or indirect financial interest in a competing entity, because nonprofit hospitals have competitive advantages including exemption from state and federal incomes taxes; exemption from sales, use, franchise, and property taxes; and the ability to raise capital through tax-exempt bonds [46].

The AMA, however, does not speak for all physicians on this issue. The American Academy of Family Physicians (AAFP) recently announced its support for extending the specialty hospital moratorium believing that specialty hospitals could cream-skim patients who have profitable diagnoses [47]. The AAFP supported continuing the moratorium until "the AAFP is convinced by evidence of their benefit on the health and well-being of our communities" [47]. The AAFP Board Chair, Michael Fleming, MD, did note, however, that the issue was not black and white. "We all have opinions about the appropriateness of this issue and whether its hurting private hospitals-particularly the safety net hospitals-to 'cherry pick.' ... Some of these specialty hospitals are actually providing excellent, very high-quality care. Some are even owned by the very hospitals that are complaining about them. So it's not a simple issue" [47].

Jean Mitchell, 2005 specialty hospital studies

Jean Mitchell is one of the prominent figures in the public relations attack against specialty and niche providers. She recently spoke before insurance professionals and employers concerned about rising health care costs at the 27th Annual Sedgwick County Health Care Roundtable Seminar held in Wichita, Kansas on October 12, 2005 [48]. The *Kansas Eagle* article that reported that Mitchell's presentation included statements that specialty hospitals turn competition in their favor and reap the financial benefits by cherry-picking patients who have less severe illnesses and cream-skimming patients who have better insurance. Specifically, self-referring physicians prescribe more ancillary services such as MRIs and physical therapy than their counterparts [48].

Additionally, Mitchell recently published "Effects of Physician-Owned Limited-Service Hospitals: Evidence from Arizona" in *Health Affairs—Web Exclusive* [49]. This article mirrors similar claims made by Mitchell in "Effects of Physician-Owned Limited Service Hospitals: Oklahoma" discussed in fuller detail later in this article. The flaws associated with Mitchell's Oklahoma study apply equally to her Arizona study.

In April 2005, the results of a study of Oklahoma physician-owned limited-service hospitals and self-referral authored by Jean M. Mitchell and entitled, "Effects of Physician-Owned Limited-Service Hospitals: Oklahoma," were published on the Website of the Coalition of Full Service Community Hospitals, http://www.fullservicehospitals.org/pdf/Research120050426.pdf, and a slide demonstration that accompanies the executive summary was published at http://www.fullservicehospitals.org/pdf/OK%20Ortho%20and%20Spine%20Hospitals_ppt.pdf.

The Mitchell's 2005 Oklahoma study analyzed data pertaining to worker's compensation claims including comparisons of the volume and use of "select orthopedic and spine procedures" across multiple facility types [50]. The 2005 Mitchell Oklahoma Study concludes that the entry of physician-owned limited-service spine and orthopedic hospitals into the Oklahoma health care market has resulted in substantial increases in the volume and use of complex spinal fusion surgery and specific orthopedic procedures, such as surgical knee replacements, non–infection-related knee procedures, and epidural pain management. Mitchell's 2005 Oklahoma study further asserts that, according to the data examined, physician-owners of select limited-service service spine and orthopedic hospitals "have steered the most profitable surgical procedures to their own facilities". Additionally, her Oklahoma study concludes that financial incentives on the part of the physician-owners in the Oklahoma City and Tulsa markets have driven this purported increase in the volume and use of inpatient complex spinal fusion surgery, outpatient pain management, outpatient removal of internal fixation devices, and non–infection related outpatient knee procedures. Mitchell claims that this asserted increase purportedly corroborates prior research findings (unidentified in the 2005 Mitchell Oklahoma study) that physician self-referral arrangements result in increased use of medical procedures and increased costs to third-party insurers.

This is not the first time that Mitchell has asserted her position against physician ownership in facilities. While employed as an Associate Professor of Economics at Florida State University, Dr. Mitchell was the Principal Investigator under a contract from the Florida Health Care Costs Containment Board for the previously described study conducted between February 1990 and August 1991 entitled, "Joint Ventures Among Health Care Providers in Florida" [51]. The purpose of this study, mandated by the Florida legislature, was "to evaluate the impact of joint ventures on access, use, costs, charges, and quality of health care services in Florida" [52]. This study was completed in 1989, the same year as a study by the Office of the Inspector General of the US Department of Health and Human Services (DHHS) related to "self-referral" arrangements for independent clinical laboratories, independent physiologic laboratories, and durable medical equipment suppliers.

The objective scientific value and validity of the 2005 Mitchell Oklahoma study, however, are significantly flawed because sample selection error and misapplication of data render the data that were collected, presented, and relied upon arbitrary, narrowly limited, and skewed as a consequence of being selectively chosen in a manner insufficient to support accurately the study's claims and conclusions. In the 2005 Mitchell Oklahoma study, empiric data cited are often cited in error, that is, without reference to modifications related to changes in certain DRG definitions, injury-reporting classifications, and other qualifications that materially affect the data submitted. These errors skew, on a fundamental level, the study's conclusions, resulting in a failure to provide any objective and reliable foundation of fact.

Combating these studies are reports such as those by the Center for Studying Health System Change (HSC). This center issued a report in June 2005 based on its Community Tracking Study in which it interviewed 95 leaders in the health care market in Indianapolis regarding the community's health system. Indianapolis, one of the 12 communities tracked by HSC every 2 years through site visits, was the basis of HSC's June report [53]. The report found the heightened development that resulted in four new heart facilities in 2002 has continued to fuel facility expansion, thereby intensifying competition among hospital systems and physicians [53]. Although the increase in competition is raising concerns about the cost of Indianapolis' health care system, Indianapolis providers are collaborating on community-wide clinical data-sharing initiatives designed to improve the quality of health care delivery, placing Indianapolis far ahead of many other communities using information technology. Most importantly, the report found, "The new heart facilities that opened in Indianapolis during the past two years have had relatively little impact on the financial performance of community hospitals to date, despite considerable fears to the contrary".

American Hospital Association case studies pressure state legislatures to impose tighter restrictions on niche providers

In addition to federal action against specialty hospitals, there have been several recent developments at the state level. The AHA argues that specialty hospitals threaten community access to basic health care services and jeopardize quality patient care. The AHA believes that allowing physicians to own hospitals leads to conflicts of interest because physicians will have a financial stake in the care provided to the patient [54]. This perceived threat to community hospitals has led to efforts to pass state legislation making it more difficult to establish specialty and niche providers.

The AHA along with the Colorado Health and Hospital Association, the Kansas Hospital Association, the Nebraska Hospital Association, and the South Dakota Association of Healthcare Organizations sponsored a study of the impact of limited-service providers on communities and full-service hospitals that was published in February 2005 [55]. The case studies found that limited-service providers had a negative impact on their communities and that they caused an increase in use and costs and concluded that physician-owners of these facilities steered their profitable patients to their own facilities [56].

Wichita, Kansas

Wichita, serving a population of approximately 1.2 million [57], saw the establishment of five physician-owned limited-service hospitals between 1999 and 2003; one heart hospital, one spine hospital, two surgical hospitals, and a joint venture between a large not-for-profit hospital and a physician group. The report found that physician-owners referred patients who had good insurance or in need of generously reimbursed procedures to their own facilities. The AHA also found that patients treated in the limited-service hospitals "tended to be in good overall health". The limited-service providers are found in Wichita's "more affluent northeast quadrant," whereas its full-service community hospitals are "located around downtown Wichita".

The report claimed a "reduction in the financial performance of the area's full-service hospitals" and "high profits at the limited-service hospitals."

Oklahoma City, Oklahoma

The study found that the limited-service hospitals generated "high profits" by focusing on the "best-paid procedures" and "patients insured by acceptable payers," resulting in "high profits and lifestyle improvements for physician owners." At the same time, full-service hospitals "declined financially" [58].

Lincoln, Nebraska

The study found that specialists shifted their patients from hospital to hospital as the specialty hospital's business strategy evolved. It documented that "many believe that health care in Lincoln is heading in the wrong direction" [59]. The study claims that the limited-service hospitals have negatively affected the community by decreasing financial resources at the full-service hospitals for low-reimbursing services such as mental health.

Black Hills region of South Dakota

Three surgical hospitals were opened in the Black Hills region between 1996 and 2000. The case study found that the use of surgical procedures in the region increased dramatically during this time. The AHA also found that the financial stability of the region's full-service hospitals declined and their bond ratings were reduced [60] and claimed that the physician-owned hospitals "achieved high profits by limiting services offered and patients served". The report also claimed that the region's full-service hospitals have been left with a "sicker mix of patients".

Missouri Hospital Association

A recent example of this public relations attack is the MHA's mass mailing of a flyer "warning" Missouri residents about the safety of "ambulatory centers" and other "limited services providers" (LSPs) with bold language such as "What You Don't Know Could Hurt You...That's Why Your Hospital Wants You to Know Some Facts About the Safety of Your Care" [61].

Through overly broad generalizations, the MHA insinuates that ASCs are under regulated. Some examples of such manipulative language include statements, such as "LSPs...are generally not subject to the same oversight and regulation," "Imaging centers and other outpatient facilities such as radiation therapy centers do not undergo comprehensive licensing and inspection by the states," and "While ambulatory surgical centers are licensed by the state, they are not held to the same level of accountability for patient safety and quality of care as hospitals."

In addition to the misleading insinuations, the MHA flyer blatantly questions the very integrity of specialty and niche providers by suggesting the Missourians should be "concerned" about such issues as whether "the center has taken precautions to assure that the instruments used to treat you are sterile an safe," whether "employees are adequately trained to assure your safety," and "will you be transferred to a facility that can provide higher levels of care should something go wrong during your procedure" [61]. Such outrageous suggestions regarding the potential lack of adequate sterilization and employee training, made by general hospitals in which thousands of deaths are caused by medical errors [62] costing millions of dollars each year, highlight the seemingly hypocritical attack by general hospitals against specialty hospital providers.

The specialty hospital regulatory environment and the effect on the transactional marketplace

The debate concerning competition for the technical component revenue streams and the surrounding turf war between physicians and hospitals greatly impacts the valuation of niche providers and physician joint ventures. The regulatory environment and the market forces driving the health care industry (which comprises one sixth of the national economy) is critical to the valuation of a health care entity. This regulatory impact is especially strong in the case of specialty hospitals and niche providers, including ASCs, which are facing increasingly strict federal and state regulations that often act as a barrier to new and competing market entrants. Specialty and niche providers often are accused of as cream-skimming or taking the more profitable cases away from general hospitals. The two facilities are reimbursed differently for the technical component of diagnostic services and surgeries. A freestanding facility is considered an office for billing purposes and is reimbursed under Medicare Part B for the technical component [63]. A hospital-based outpatient department with provider-based status is reimbursed for the technical component under Medicare Part A [64]. In light of these attacks and the uncertain regulatory future, it is imperative that physicians understand both the public relations attacks and the regulatory threats to their business relationships and joint ventures.

The valuation of specialty providers, even more than of other health care providers, promises to continue to be heavily influenced by technological and competitive factors. Continuing technological advances in diagnostic and therapeutic equipment may further increase the competitive pressures between hospitals and physicians for technical component revenue streams. Competition over the technical component revenue streams and the regulatory uncertainty affecting specialty and niche providers intrinsically drive up the risk of participating in health care transactions involving these providers.

History, definition, and trends of specialty and niche providers

The recent attacks against specialty hospitals, although widely publicized, are not new. The federal government began controlling the business practices of physicians through a complex scheme of legislative and regulatory activities [65]. Against the backdrop of the perceived threat stemming from the growth of specialty and niche providers, it is of paramount importance to emphasize that the United States has a long tradition of niche providers [66]. There is an extensive history of specialty hospitals such as rehabilitation hospitals, children's hospitals, cancer hospitals, and psychiatric hospitals. The distinguishing characteristic of specialty hospitals subjected to the recent intense governmental scrutiny is the ownership interests of the physicians who refer patients to them [65]. Thus, the issue seems to be merely a result of general hospitals' attempt to prevent competition and limit the entry of specialty hospitals into the health care marketplace.

Historical changes to the balance of power between the profession of medicine and hospitals and resulting definitions of specialty and niche providers

"Limited-service providers, also known as 'niche' or specialty providers are not new, but the nature and pace of their growth is" [67]. The existence of surgical hospitals is not a new idea. Specialty hospitals for children, rehabilitation, and diseases of the eye and ear have a long-established, celebrated history in the United States, but hospitals focusing on cardiovascular and orthopedic procedures are relatively new. In recent years, in response to market dynamics and the desire to exert more control over their own clinical services to patients, some specialists have entered into joint ventures with majority-owner non-physician investors to build single-specialty hospitals such as surgical, orthopedic, spine, and cardiac hospitals.

These providers have been variously defined to include ASCs, surgical hospitals, specialty hospitals, and a host of other narrowly focused providers. Healthcare providers falling into the broad category termed "niche" providers focus on a section or group of buyers, a segment of a product line, or a specific area of a geographic market. The AHA broadly defines niche providers to include "heart hospitals, orthopedic hospitals, surgical hospitals, ASCs, cancer hospitals and centers, dialysis clinics, pain centers, imaging centers, mammography centers, and a host of other narrowly focused providers" [68]. The AHA, however, does not include other types of specialty and niche services such as trauma and intensive care, which require extensive specialization and are provided solely within the traditional inpatient hospital setting.

To evaluate the attack on specialty and niche providers, this term may be defined broadly to include any health care provider who provides a specialized level of care and/or medical treatment outside a traditional inpatient hospital setting. Such providers include ASCs that perform surgical procedures on an outpatient basis, surgical and specialty hospitals, and all health care providers that might be affected by attempts to prohibit physician investment in facilities and medical equipment. A broad, inclusive definition of specialty and niche providers, such as that developed by the AHA, is necessary because nontraditional health care providers increasingly compete with traditional health care providers.

In search of the threat from specialty and niche providers

Although the hospital industry's attack on specialty and niche providers is motivated by fear of the competition these providers bring to the market, the attacks usually are framed in terms of the threat these providers pose to the public interest. Duplication of services once again has seized center stage in the media commentary of the changing health care delivery system in the United States. Administrators from existing general acute-care hospital systems and their supporters have led the hue and cry against what they claim to be duplication. Their fixation on duplication stems from a seemingly misguided and misinformed assertion that societal costs increase when there are "too many" providers of the same health services—a situation labeled as "excess capacity."

"Excess capacity," however, is a value-laden term, not an absolute standard. In a recent article published in *Health Services Research* (February 1999), Carolyn Madden summarized a number of studies of excess capacity, saying, "Without a clear statement of this standard [eg, the correct number of hospital beds], we cannot determine what constitutes too many. The research literature provides no clear statement" [69]. The trouble with duplication is that everyone seems to be against it, but nobody knows what it means. The debate can be characterized as an argument about "whose ox gets gored."

On the topic of duplication, independent physicians often have been called "cherry-pickers." The implication is that these physicians are greedy, and their business is inconsistent with maximizing community health. This designation probably dismisses the importance of patient choice and seems to proceed with a one-dimensional focus on market monopoly. The ideal health care delivery system seeks value by considering all the important components: access, quality, beneficial outcomes, appropriate cost, and patient choice. For patient choice to exist, there must be more than one service provider, because choice, by definition, involves alternatives. Duplication, by definition, is the existence of more than one service provider. Thus, arguments against duplication are arguments against patient choice.

New facilities (whether developed from the ground up or remodeled from existing facilities) are being built. This process is inevitable and desirable. Modern facilities accommodate innovative technologies and protocols that provide higher-quality care and operate at a lower cost per square foot. The real concern about duplication involves the control of the new facilities. Patients have a right to choose their own independent physicians at convenient locations. Let the quality of services and beneficial outcomes define the level of competition, not the politics of power.

CON or similar programs, in which the government determines where, when, and how capital expenditures will be made for health care facilities and major equipment, shield existing providers from competition. Michael Morrisey of the University of Alabama-Birmingham Center for Health Policy argues that established providers will fight to influence public policy to shelter themselves from competition and maintain market leverage with payers and patients. Morrisey suggests that CON laws are resurfacing in some states to protect existing hospitals from competition and, in turn, are decreasing pressure to reduce capacity and prices [70]. When that happens, incentives to improve quality decrease as well. The fundamental, but flawed, idea offered by many CON proponents was simple: lower costs by reducing duplication. Economic and health care scholars, however, concluded that CON laws were a miserable failure. In an article reviewing the CON law and its application to modern markets, Patrick J. McGinley wrote, "In searching the scholarly journals, one cannot find a single article that asserts that CON laws succeed in lowering health care costs" [69].

Research observation and findings

There have been several studies on the effect of surgical and specialty hospitals on the competitive marketplace. Some studies have been conducted by private for-profit contractors such as the Lewin Group. Other studies have been conducted by the government, sometimes at the prompting and lobbying of general hospitals and groups such as the AHA [71]. Thus, even studies conducted by the government that seem to be impartial may be influenced through the lobbying by general hospital groups in conjunction with the government's own financial interests and motives.

In response to the highly suspect earlier studies by interested parties and those conducted by private for-profit contractors, Health Capital Consultants conducted its own study on the effect, if any, that the presence of a surgical hospital in a market had on the financial "health" of the general, acute-care hospitals in the market. The Health Capital Consultants analysis indicated that there is not a significant difference between the profit margins on either a per bed or a per admission basis of general, acute-care hospitals in metropolitan statistical areas with a surgical hospital and those in metropolitan statistical areas without a surgical hospital.

Government Accountability Office reports

The GAO released its study, "Specialty Hospitals: Information on National Market Share, Physician Ownership, and Patients Served" in April 2003. This study examined the share of the national market comprising specialty hospitals and determined that, as of February 2003, the 92 cardiac, orthopedic, surgical, and women's hospitals identified accounted for less than 2% of short-term acute-care hospitals nationwide. The study analyzed the extent to which physicians had ownership interests in specialty hospitals and determined that about 70% of specialty hospitals in existence or under development had some physician ownership. Among these hospitals, total physician ownership averaged slightly more than 50%. Additionally, the study compared patients served by specialty hospitals with those served by general hospitals in terms of illness severity and concluded that patients at specialty hospitals tend to be less sick than patients who have the same diagnosis at general hospitals.

In October 2003 the GAO released its second study, "Specialty Hospitals: Geographic Location, Services Provided, and Financial Performance." This study examined the extent to which specialty hospitals are clustered in areas where state policy and local demographic conditions favor growth and analyzed the degree to which specialty hospitals rivaled general hospitals in certain market-share measures and financial performance. The study concluded that the number of specialty hospitals is growing rapidly, with an expected 25% increase within the months following the issuance of the study, that specialty hospitals are among the larger competitors facing general hospitals, and that the economic impact of specialty hospitals on general hospitals remains unknown.

US Department of Health and Human Services 2005 report

In addition to the MedPAC study, the Medicare Act of 2003 required a study to be performed related to specialty and surgical hospitals by the US Department of Health and Human Services (DHHS). In March 2005, the DHHS reported several significant findings. The report stated

> Specialty hospitals provide a high level of quality of care. From the site visits and focus groups we found that structural measures of quality, such as staff specialization and clinical staff per patient, suggest a high quality of care in this dimension. In addition, process of care measures, such as complication rates, also suggest good performance on the part of specialty hospitals. Except for the higher readmission rates, outcome measures such as, mortality rates, discharge disposition all suggest that the patients treated at specialty hospitals experience a high quality of care [72].

The study suggested that patients highly value the amenities, such as a quiet environment, private rooms, accessibility and attentiveness of a specialized nursing staff, and specialized treatments and procedures, because these factors contribute to their recovery. The study further indicated that patients view physician ownership as way to improve physician attentiveness because of their personal stake in the specialty hospitals.

University of Iowa study

The American Surgical Hospital Association, the association representing the surgical hospital industry, commissioned researchers at the University of Iowa to conduct an independent study of the impact of surgical hospitals on health care markets. The study, "Economics and Policy Analysis of Specialty Hospitals," was directed by John E. Schneider, PhD, University of Iowa [73].

The study found economic advantages associated with specialization, resulting mainly from process redesign, learning, avoidance of diseconomies of scope, and focus on core competencies. Specialty hospitals seem to have patient outcomes equal to or better than outcomes in their general hospital counterparts [73]. Additionally, the study found that because specialty hospitals compete with general hospitals in the same manner in which general hospitals compete with each other, there was no evidence to suggest that general hospitals have been harmed financially by competition from specialty hospitals or that such competition is undesirable from a societal perspective [73]. Finally, the study found no evidence that physician self-referral is a problem in specialty hospitals for four reasons: (1) the majority of studies of higher use resulting from self-referral are based on physician ownership in ancillary services; (2) there is no direct evidence that that self-referral is motivated by disproportionate financial incentives; (3) there is no direct evidence that physician self-referrals result in worse outcomes; and (4) in the case of physician ownership of acute-care facilities, it is likely that the magnitude of financial incentives is limited [73].

Federal Trade Commission and Department of Justice hearings on health care and competition law and policy

In November 2002, FTC Chairman Timothy J. Muris, announced that the FTC would hold joint hearings with the DOJ on competition in health care in 2003 [74]. On July 23, 2004, following the conclusion of the hearings lasting more than 6 months, the FTC and DOJ issued a joint report on July 23, 2004, entitled "Improving Health Care: A Dose of Competition" in which the agencies recommended that states decrease barriers to entry into provider markets. The agencies encouraged states to reconsider whether CON programs "best serve their citizens' health care needs". Following testimony at numerous hearings from industry representatives and legal, economic, and academic experts on the health care industry and health policy, the agencies concluded that the burdens placed on competition by CON programs "generally outweigh" its "purported economic benefits" and suggested that, instead of reducing costs, CON programs actually may increase costs by "fostering anticompetitive barriers to entry".

The agencies expressed concern that CON programs raise health care costs because they seem to depress supply and protect health care providers from competition. The agencies were concerned further that CON programs tend to prevent entry into the market by entities that seem to be able to provide higher quality care and contended that CON programs may delay the introduction of new technology. In support of their conclusions, the agencies relied upon empiric studies that showed CON programs generally failed to control costs and actually seemed to result in higher health care costs. In response to allegations by ASC providers that general hospitals have attempted to use CON laws to prevent ASCs from entering the market, the agencies committed to "aggressively pursuing" activities of anticompetitive conduct while acknowledging that antitrust laws do not prevent individual hospitals from unilaterally approaching state governments in connection with CON proceedings.

The report also summarized the controversy surrounding competition by surgical and specialty hospitals (SSHs). "A recently imposed Congressional moratorium on physician referrals to SSHs in which they have an ownership interest and two Congressionally mandated studies on SSHs and general hospitals will likely affect the future of SSHs" [75]. At the same time, the report recommends, "States should decrease barriers to entry into provider markets". A further observation is that

> Private parties should not engage in anticompetitive conduct in responding to marketplace developments. ...The permissibility of unilateral and collective provider conduct in response to marketplace developments (including P4P tiering, SSHs, and ASCs) is raised in several different settings in the Report. ... If there is specific evidence of anticompetitive conduct by individual providers or provider collusion in response to marketplace developments, the Agencies will aggressively pursue those activities.

In light of these FTC pronouncements, it remains to be seen what impact this report will actually have on the continuing existence or enforcement of state CON legislation. Nonetheless, this federal report is, perhaps, the most significant development in the last several years in the ongoing battle to eliminate CON and support a level playing field for market competition in health care.

Summary

Understanding the evolving and increasingly expansive definitions of "specialty hospitals," "niche providers," and "limited-service providers" is crucial for understanding how these various providers and facilities compete and are being subjected to attack in the form of increasing legislation and regulation affecting physician ownership and other financial relationships with these facilities. The attack on specialty and niche providers, currently expanded to comprise what the AHA terms "limited-service providers," now threatens to stifle competition, halt innovation, and divert attention away from hospital's legitimate quality and charity care problems.

These recent attacks have again raised accusations of conflict of interest for physician-owners who refer patients to surgical hospitals in which they have an ownership interest. The inference is that physicians may not be trusted to make clinical decisions and that they would refer patients for unnecessary surgeries. There is growing evidence, however, that physicians provide higher-quality medical care with more beneficial outcomes and are better able to meet patient demands when physicians have both operational control and a financial stake in the facilities where they are providing care to their patients [76]. Any reasonable interpretation of the motives underlying these attacks must conclude that the attacks have nothing to do with quality of care and patient safety but rather are a pre-emptive strike to limit competition.

Hospitals have claimed that they need to be overpaid to shift costs to support their emergency rooms, ICUs, 24-hour service, charity care, and generally sicker patients [5]. These claims were made despite a drop in hospitals' charity care (as a percent of expenses) in 2003 to its lowest level since 1983. The year 2003 was also the first year since 1980 that expenditures for charity care were lower than in the previous year [77]. General hospital groups often have cited the development of ASCs and surgical hospitals as the cause of declining general hospitals finances and also of general hospital closures. The annual number of hospitals closures declined between 1987 and 1994, however, years in which the number of ASCs more than doubled [78]. Numerous other factors have been cited as causes for the decline in hospitals nationally, including the following:

1. The excess bed capacity of hospitals during the enormous shift from inpatient to outpatient care
2. Failure to adjust to managed care and large reductions in average length of stay
3. Hospital mergers and acquisitions leading to large-scale market consolidation, including closure of facilities, during the 1990s
4. The costly failure of vertical integration efforts, including the acquisition of physician practices

A 2002 analysis of data through 1999 related to two selected markets in which physician-owned ASCs were developed showed ambiguous results for local hospitals. Generally, after an initial drop in surgical volume, both the ASC and the local hospital resumed earlier growth trends.

> Combined with the well-documented shift of medical care from an inpatient to an outpatient setting, the rise in physician-owned facilities has placed heavy competitive pressure on acute care hospitals. Hospitals have responded to that pressure by pushing back, in one fashion or another. The resultant collisions have sparked antitrust lawsuits in which the conduct of the physician-owned facility (the new entrant) is cast as the force for competition, while the conduct of the hospital (the established incumbent) is cast as the force against competition. This intuitive characterization is undoubtedly apt in many instances; no competitor applauds the launch of a new rival, and an incumbent's responses to new entry may include suppressing rather than adapting to the new competition [79].

General hospitals often accuse physician-investors of self-referral, cream-skimming, and cherry-picking. Every service line in general acute-care hospitals, with the possible exception of trauma care and ICUs, is subject to competition, perhaps by physicians and freestanding providers but most certainly by other general hospitals, assuming that the hospitals have not eliminated that competition by forming a monopoly or oligopoly. General acute-care hospitals do not have to perform these non-trauma care services any more than licensed general acute-care hospitals that specialize in surgery or other specialties are required to perform certain specific non-trauma care service lines.

If costs are to be controlled and quality maintained through competitive forces, there must be a level playing field for competitors. Hospital lobbies are attempting to outlaw their competition rather than to create a level playing field on which to compete. If there were a rational, empirically based indication that hospital outpatient procedures are reimbursed at too high a level, the government should restructure the payments to emergency care and intensive care services. Similarly, if reimbursement for certain surgical and specialty procedures is too high, payment should be adjusted and funds redirected to emergency and intensive care services (if they actually are underfunded).

If physicians do not ensure that there is a freely competitive market, there are only two alternatives. The first is to allow general acute-care hospitals to be shielded from competition and thus from the market incentives that result in lower costs and improvements in quality by fostering innovation. This situation generally is regarded as unfair and undesirable. The second alternative is to provide health care as a government service similar to the national defense and space programs. Most would agree that neither of these solutions is in the best interest of patients, payors, providers, or the federal and state governments.

Specialty and niche providers are so diverse a group that they have little overall cohesiveness. In addition, the various medical specialties have been split because of the differing interests of primary care physicians versus specialists and other conflicts. The AHA, however, considers limited-service providers as a single group including "heart hospitals, orthopedic hospitals, surgical hospitals, ASCs, cancer hospitals and centers, dialysis clinics, pain centers, imaging centers, mammography centers, and a host of other narrowly focused providers". Specialty and niche providers must come together, unified by the well-organized and coordinated threat to their very existence. Only with a unified and coordinated effort, through their respective associations, will specialty and niche providers be effective in their fight against hospitals' desire to monopolize technical component revenue streams.

Leading health care economist Michael Porter has identified three generic strategies to outperform competitors or maintain a market position against competition: overall cost leadership, differentiation, and market niche/segmentation. The last, market niche/segmentation, as discussed earlier, recognizes the competitive legitimacy of competition based on focusing on a single market niche or segment, as health care specialty and niche providers have done. This approach allows them to create "focused factories" that have been demonstrated to improve quality and efficiency, thereby benefiting consumers. Michael Porter [80] has further stated:

> In industry after industry, the underlying dynamic is the same: competition compels companies to deliver increasing value to customers. The fundamental driver of this continuous quality improvement and cost reduction is innovation. Without incentives to sustain innovation in health care, short-term cost savings will soon be overwhelmed by the desire to widen access, the growing health needs of an aging population, and the unwillingness of Americans to settle for anything less than the best treatments available. Inevitably, the failure to promote innovation will lead to lower quality or more rationing of care—two equally undesirable results.

The issues documented in this article continue to frame the battle between physicians and hospitals. Who should control and profit from technical component revenue streams from procedures and diagnostic testing is at its heart a turf war between physicians and hospitals. The appropriate option is to remove the market barriers to innovation and allow "the better mousetrap" to prevail.

References

[1] Improving health care: a dose of competition. Washington, DC: Department of Justice and Federal Trade Commission; 2004.

[2] Healthgrades. Patient safety in American hospitals. Available at: www.healthgrades.com/media/english/pdf/HG_Patient_Safety_Study_Final.pdf. Accessed March 2, 2005.

[3] American Hospital Association. Impact of physician-owned limited-service hospitals: Oklahoma City Case Study. Chicago, Feb. 16, 2005. p. 22.

[4] Ambulatory surgery centers' Medicare pay rate questioned. AMedNews.com. Nov. 2, 2002. Available at: http://www.ama-assn.org/sci-pubs/amnews/pick_02/gvsa1125.htm. Accessed May 20, 2003.

[5] Hospitals cry foul: HHS report urges reimbursement adjustments. Mod Healthc 2003;10.

[6] This just in: MedPAC proposal likely won't make Medicare bill. Outpatient Surgery Aug. 2003. Available at: http://www.outpatientsurgery.net/2003/os08/news.php. Accessed October 1, 2003.

[7] Connolly C. Tax-exempt hospitals' practices challenged. Washington Post. January 29, 2005:A1.

[8] Kohn LT, Corrigan J, Donaldson M. (Committee on Quality Health Care in America, Institute of Medicine) To err is human: building a safer health system. Washington, DC: National Academy Press 1999. p. 1.

[9] Infection epidemic carves deadly path. Chicago Tribune. July 21, 2002:1.

[10] New push after transplant tragedy—hospitals search for ways to prevent errors, help doctors learn from others. Doctorquality. Available at: http://www.doctorquality.com/www/products/rpm/resources/news_022003.htm. Accessed October 1, 2003.

[11] Med complications may cost $9B per year. Yahoo! News. Oct. 7, 2003. Available at: news.yahoo.com/news?tmpl=story2&cid=534&u=/ap/2003100//

ap_on_he_me/costly_complications&printer=1. Accessed October 8, 2003.

[12] Kwiecinski M. Limiting conflicts of interest arising from physician investment in specialty hospitals. Marquette Law Review 2004;88:417.

[13] Federal Trade Commission and Department of Justice. Hearings on health care and competition law and policy [transcript]. Available at: http://www.ftc.gov/ogc/healthcarehearings/030326ftctrans.pdf. Accessed November 16, 2007.

[14] Medicare Prescription Drug, Modernization, Improvement Act of 2003,§507(a)(1)(B).

[15] US General Accounting Office. Specialty hospitals: information on national market share, physician ownership, and patients served. US General Accounting Office, Apr. 18, 2003. p. 3, 8.

[16] US Government Accountability Office. Specialty hospital moratorium. GAO-05–647R: 3, 6, 7. Washington, DC: US General Accounting Office May 19, 2005.

[17] Romano M. Specialty hospital ban ends, debate continues. Available at: http://www.modernhealthcare.com.

[18] Gordon J. Moratorium on specialty hospitals expires. Dallas Business Journal June, 20, 2005. Available at: http://www.bizjournals.com/dallas/stories/2005/06/20/story8.html. Accessed November 2007.

[19] Barr P, Becker C, Benko LB, et al. Outlook 2005: money, money, money. Mod Healthc 2005;35(1):26.

[20] Specialty hospitals. Environmental assessment. 2005. Available at: http://ea.acponline.org/systems/SH.html. Accessed October 11, 2005.

[21] Glendinning D. Medicare pay freeze not yet final, but likely. Amednews.com. January 2, 2006. Available at: http://www.ama-assn.org/amednews/2006/01/02/gvl10102.htm. Accessed January 9, 2006.

[22] Director of Centers for Medicare and Medicaid Services Survey and Certification Group. Hospitals—suspension of processing new provider enrollment applications (CMS-855A) for specialty hospitals. Chicago: Centers for Medicare & Medicaid Services; 2005.

[23] Testimony of Mark B. McClellan, MD, Ph.D., administrator, Centers for Medicare & Medicaid Services, before the House Committee. May 14, 2005. Available at: http://www.cms.hhs.gov/apps/media/press/testimony.asp?Counter=1459. Accessed January 9, 2006.

[24] Senate Bill 1884. 2005; House Bill 4202. 2005.

[25] Summary of the Ambulatory Surgical Center Payment Modernization Act. Available at: http://aaasc.org/documents/ASCModernizationActSummaryandFacts92305_000.doc. Accessed October 21, 2005.

[26] Article highlights self-referral concerns, senators say [editorial]. AHA News Now. August 9, 2005. Available at: http://www.ahanews.com/ahanews_app/hospitalconnect/search/article.jsp?dcrpath=AHANEWS/AHANewsNowArticle/data/ann_050809_Grassley&domain=AHANEWS.

[27] Grassley C, Bauccus M. Letter to Senate re Washington Post editorial on specialty hospital referral, August 9, 2005. Hospital Fair Competition Act of 2005. S. 1002, 109th Congress, 1st Session May 11, 2005.

[28] American Hospital Association. Bill proposes permanent ban on specialty hospitals. June 13, 2005. Available at: www.hospitalconnet.com. Accessed September 15, 2005.

[29] Fong T. CMS asked to review specialty hospitals for racial bias [letter to CMS Administrator Mark McClellan. July 28, 2005]. Modern Physician [serial online]. Available at: http://www.modernphysician.com/printwindow.cms?newsId=3834&pageType=news. Accessed August 29, 2005.

[30] MedPAC.Report to the Congress. Physician-owned specialty hospitals. Washington, DC: Medicare Payment Advisory Commission; 2005. p. 7, 8, 17.

[31] Thompson T. Self-referral issue isolates radiology in multispecialty forum. Auntminnie. October 7, 2004. Available at: www.auntminnie.com/index.asp?Sec=sup&Sub=imc&Pag=dis&ItemID=63177. Accessed February 18, 2005.

[32] Volkin L, Dargan R. Self-referral drives increase in diagnostic imaging among nonradiologists. American Society of Radiologic Technologists December 10, 2004; Available at: www.asrt.org/content/News/IndustryNewsBrief/GenRes/Selfreferr041210.aspx. Accessed February 18, 2005.

[33] Bricc J. ACR pursues designated physician imager legislation. Diagnostic Imaging [serial online] 2005; Available at: www.diagnosticimagingonline/showNews.jhtml?articleID=577700160 Accessed February 18, 2005.

[34] Medicare Payment Advisory Commission. Transcript of public meeting. Washington, DC: Medicare Payment Advisory Commission; 2004. p. 295–6.

[35] American College of Radiology. Accreditation. Available at: http://www.acr.org/s_acr/sec.asp?CID=2541&DID=17586. Accessed May 9, 2005.

[36] Taylor M. System dumps doc investors in specialty hospital. Mod healthc [serial online] 2004; Available at: www.modernphysician.com/printwindow.cms?newsId=1710&pageType=news. Accessed February 15, 2004.

[37] Weeks E. The new economic credentialing: protecting hospitals from competition by medical staff members. J Health Law 2003;36:247.

[38] Lister v Methodist Medical Center of Oak Ridge, 1993. WL 481402.

[39] Fair Trade Commission/Department of Justice. Hearings on hospital competition focus on specialty hospitals, contracting. BNA Health Law Reporter News. 2003;12:513.

[40] New Jersey Assembly Bill No. 3127.

[41] Medical Society of New Jersey. MSNJ opposes A-3127 tax on ambulatory care centers [press release]. Medical Society of New Jersey, Lawrenceville, NJ, June 22, 2004.

[42] Norbut M. New taxes in New Jersey target doctor services. American Medical Association. 2004. Available at: www.ama-assn.org/amednews/2004/09/13/bisb0913.htm. Accessed February 25, 2005.

[43] Limited service providers: an overview. Missouri Hospital Association. 2005. Available at: web.mhanet.com/asp/Governmental_Relations/state_advocacy/limited_service_providers.asp. Accessed February 23, 2005.

[44] Open heart surgery/certificates of need. Florida HB 329. 2004.

[45] Betbeze P. ASCs sellouts or saviors. HealthLeaders. October 2004. Available at: www.healthleaders.com/magazine/cover.php?contentid=58684. Accessed March 1, 2005.

[46] Maves M. Ambulatory surgery center, and general hospitals: charting wise public policy. Presentation to the Council on Health Care Economics and Policy on Specialty Hospitals. Sept. 10, 2004. Available at: http://council.brandeis.edu/pubs/Specialty%20Hospitals/Maves%20Presentation.pdf. Accessed November 2007.

[47] Extend moratorium on specialty hospitals says board. American Academy of Family Physicians, 2005. Available at: www.aafp.org/x31982.xml. Accessed February 28, 2005.

[48] Atwater A. Do doctor-owned hospitals drive up health care costs? The Wichita Eagle October 13, 2005; section 4:B.

[49] Mitchell J. Effects of physician-owned limited-service hospitals: evidence from Arizona. Health affairs Web exclusive. 2005. Available at: http://www.healthaffairs.org/. Accessed October 16, 2005.

[50] Mitchell J. Effects of physician-owned limited-service spine and orthopedic hospitals. Washington, DC: Georgetown University Public Policy Institute; 2005. p. 3–5.

[51] Curriculum vitae: Jean M. Mitchell. Georgetown University. Available at: www.georgetown.edu/faculty/mitchell.html. Accessed May 25, 2005.

[52] Joint ventures among health care providers in Florida. State of Florida Health Care Cost Containment Board. Tallahasee, FL, September 1991;2;ii.

[53] Continued hospital expansion raise cost concerns in Indianapolis. Community Report No. 2 of 12. Washington, DC: Center for Studying Health System Change; June 2005. p. 1, 2.

[54] American Hospital Association. Perspectives on competition policy and health care marketplace: single specialty hospitals. Statement before the Department of Justice and Federal Trade Commission Hearing March 27, 2003. American Hospital Association. Available at: http://www.aha.org/aha/testimony/2003/030227-tesvarney-doj-ftc.html. Accessed November 2007.

[55] American Hospital Association. Special studies and reports. Available at: www.hospitalconnect.com/aha/press_room-info/specialstudies.html. Accessed March 1, 2005.

[56] The impact of physician-owned limited-service hospitals: a summary of four case studies. American Hospital Association, Feb. 16, 2005. Available at: www.aha.org/aha/key_issues/niche/content/050207summary.pdf. Accessed February 28, 2005.

[57] American Hospital Association. Impact of physician-owned limited-service hospitals. Wichita, KS case study. Chicago: American Hospital Association; 2005. p. 2, 3, 5, 8.

[58] American Hospital Association. Impact of physician-owned limited-service hospitals. Oklahoma City case study. Chicago: American Hospital Association; 2005. p. 3.

[59] American Hospital Association. Impact of physician-owned limited-service hospitals. Lincoln case study. Chicago: American Hospital Association; 2005. p. 3, 17.

[60] American Hospital Association. Impact of physician-owned limited-service hospitals. Black Hills case study. Nov. 18, 2004. p. 2, 6, 19.

[61] Missouri Hospital Association. What you don't know could hurt you [Flyer mailed to Missouri citizens]. Jefferson City, MO: Missouri Hospital Association; 2005.

[62] See study patient safety in American hospitals. Health grades quality study: patient safety in American hospitals. Healthgrades. July, 2004. Available at: www.healthgrades.com/media/english/pdf/HG_Patient_Safety_Study_Final.pdf. Accessed March 2, 2005.

[63] ECG Management Consultants. Provider-based clinics. Despite APCs and stricter clinic requirements, financial opportunities remain. ECG Management Consultants. Available at: http://www.ecgmc.com/insights_ideas/pdfs/Provider-Based_Clinics_Financial_Opportunities.pdf.

[64] Nycomed Amersham Imaging. Radiation oncology reimbursement reference guide. 2000. Available at: www.us-nai.com/reimb/Radiation%20Oncology%20MCR%20B%20Explained.htm. Accessed March 13, 2003.

[65] Iglehart J. The emergence of physician-owned specialty hospitals. N Engl J Med 2005;352:78.

[66] Devers K. Specialty hospitals: focused factories or cream skimmers? Center for Studying Health System Change Health System Issue Brief No. 62. Washington, DC: Center for Studying Health System Change; 2003.

[67] Limited service – niche providers. American Hospital Association. 2005. Available at: www.hospitalconnect.com/aha/key_issues/niche/. Accessed February 27, 2005.

[68] Promises under pressure. American Hospital Association. Available at: www.hospitalconnect.com/aha/annual_meeting/content/03mtgpaper_Niche.pdf. Accessed February 27, 2005.

[69] McGinley JP. Beyond health care reform: reconsidering certificate of need laws in a managed care completion system. Florida State University Law Review 1995;23:141–88.

[70] Madden CW. Excess capacity: markets, regulation, and values. Health Services Research. February 1999;33:1669–82.
[71] Iglehart J. The emergence of physician-owned specialty hospitals. N Engl J Med 2005;352:83–4.
[72] Levitt MO. Study of physician-owned specialty hospitals required in Section 507(c)(2) of the Medicare Prescription Drug, Improvement, and Modernization Act of 2003. Washington, DC: Centers for Medicare and Medicaid Services; 2005. p. 48–54.
[73] Schneider JE. Economics and policy analysis of specialty hospitals. HECG. Available at: (http://www.surgicalhospital.org/pdfs/HECG_Final_Report.pdf). Accessed February 4, 2005.
[74] Federal Trade Commission. FTC chairman announces public hearings on health care and competition law and policy to begin in February 2003. Available at: www.ftc.gov/opa/2002/11/muris healthcare.htm. Accessed August 5, 2004.
[75] American Medical Association. Conflicts of interest: health facility ownership by a physician. Journal of the American Medical Association 1992;267:2366–9.
[76] Casalino LP, Devers KJ, Brewster LR, et al. Focused factories? Physician owned specialty facilities. Health Aff 2003;22:56–67.
[77] Charitable dropoff. Uncompensated care drops to lowest level in years. Mod Healthc 2003:4.
[78] Does ambulatory surgery center development cause hospital closures? Outpatient Surgery. October, 1997:1–2.
[79] Lynk WJ, Longley CS. The effect of physician-owned surgicenters on hospital outpatient surgery. Health Aff 2002;21:215–21.
[80] Teisberg EO, Porter M, Brown GB, et al. Making competition in health care work. Harv Bus Rev 1994;72:131–42.

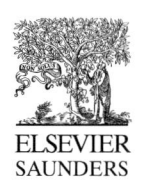

Making the Electronic Medical Record Work for the Orthopedic Surgeon

Louis F. McIntyre, MD

Westchester Orthopedic Associates, 222 Westchester Avenue, Suite 101, White Plains, NY 10604, USA

The health care industry in the United States is a huge information business that accounts for $1.7 trillion per year in economic activity. There is a national discussion concerning the rising cost, inefficiency, and human error in the system and methods of solving these vexing and complex problems. Many industries in the United States have seen impressive gains in productivity leading to greater value with the application of computer technology in processing the information necessary to conduct business. Information technology (IT) is credited with between one third to one fourth of the 6% to 8% productivity gains seen per year in the telecommunications, securities trading, and retail merchandising sectors of the economy [1]. What if the health care industry could realize similar productivity increases with the widespread application of computer technology in the form of an electronic medical record (EMR)? Recently, senior management scientists at the RAND Corporation tried to answer this question and estimated that, with 90% adoption of IT throughout both the inpatient and outpatient portions of the health care system, yearly savings could be $77 billion per year! Theoretically, these savings would come from decreased length of hospital stay, reduced nursing and physician administration time, reduced drug and radiology usage, and prevention of error, addressing many of the issues that plague the system. The authors cite the additional benefits of using IT for short-term preventive care and long-term chronic disease management [2]. Many believe that the widespread application of IT to health care will not only help but will solve the system's problems [1–6].

Because the federal treasury pays for almost 50% of all health care delivered in the United States, government policy experts look at such potential savings with great interest. Across the political spectrum, from Hillary Clinton to Newt Gingrich, EMR is seen as a panacea for the problems that afflict the system [7], President George Bush mentioned the adoption of EMRs in his State of the Union messages in 2004 and 2006. In 2003 the Department of Health and Human Services asked the Institute of Medicine to provide guidance concerning the capabilities of EMR systems. The report predicted that widespread regional use of a standardized EMR system will become a reality by 2010 [3]. There is no clear plan to implement or pay for this transition, despite significant public sector interest in a migration to electronic record keeping.

Although there may be macroeconomic benefits to system-wide use of EMR, most doctors live in the microeconomic world of private practice in small to medium-sized groups [8].

As a result, most doctors look at the decision to purchase an EMR strictly from a business perspective and consider return on investment more important than decreasing health care spending or quality improvement. This article explores the current reasons why orthopedic surgeons might consider the adoption of an EMR in their practices today. The costs and benefits as well as the barriers to implementation are discussed.

The structure and function of the medical record

Medicine is an information industry dedicated to the acquisition and management of data, but the medical record has been a marginalized

E-mail address: lfm@woapc.com

portion of physician training and attention. Generating, storing, and analyzing medical records are the least favorite tasks of practicing physicians and surgeons. The irony is that they are one of the most important and potentially valuable functions physicians perform. It therefore is appropriate to define what the medical record is, its form, and what it is supposed to accomplish.

The medical record currently serves three purposes. First, it stores information used by providers and coordinates medical care. Second, it provides legal documentation of the physician–patient interaction for the purposes of litigation. Third, Medicare and insurance companies use the medical record to determine the appropriate level of physician reimbursement. In an information age, the medical record has become an extremely important source of health, legal, and economic data. To be useful to an orthopedic practice, an electronically generated record must fulfill all of these functions while decreasing operating costs and enhancing office workflow to increase productivity and truly to add value [4].

An EMR must be clear and concise but contain the pertinent clinical data that surgeons are familiar with in traditional medical record keeping. The format of the clinical part of the record should resemble the outline that most surgeons recognize, with headings for subjective history, objective findings, assessment of the problem, and a plan for treatment. The EMR should be well organized and easy to read. The record should be comprehensive, with modules for storage and retrieval of diagnostic tests, surgical images, and scanning of correspondences and other clerical materials. The record should be transmissible between different practitioners in both the same and different medical specialties with the expectation that each will understand the information transmitted without ambiguity. In addition, the record should be secure to protect patient confidentiality.

The EMR is a legal document and as such must satisfy the needs of the legal system in documenting the physician–patient relationship. The record should contain all the pertinent positive and negative findings germane to the patient's problem and document issues of informed consent and patient education. All aspects of physician–patient interaction must be contained in the record, from office visits to hospital consultations and telephone calls. It must be flexible enough to reflect the complexity that individual patients present to physicians. It cannot be a liability for patients or physicians when problems arise.

Last, the record must satisfy the current Evaluation and Management (E&M) coding guidelines [9]. The guidelines fix set codes to certain levels of documentation of care. As a result, the medical record is essential in determining the appropriate level of reimbursement. The guidelines must be followed to avoid the accusation of Medicare or insurance fraud in billing practices and to ensure that orthopedic practitioners are reimbursed properly. It is helpful, therefore, to have the structure of the record mimic the guidelines and their headings of chief complaint, history of present illness, review of systems, past medical and social history, physical findings, imaging studies, treatments, and medical decision-making complexity.

The structure of the electronic record has three main components. The first is the demographic and billing component that most orthopedic offices already possess and understand. The second is the application that allows the creation of an office note with the attributes previously described. The third is the program that takes the place of the paper chart and stores all the information previously mentioned plus any paper or electronic correspondence that comes to the office. The second component is most often referred to as the "EMR." This is the program that the surgeon must use to enter and retrieve clinical data pertaining to the history and physical examination. The EMR alone does not accomplish the goal of a paperless environment; the addition of an electronic chart completes the transition to a truly electronic health record. The electronic chart component facilitates the retrieval of patient information by storing it in digital folders that hold all data in an organized format. The electronic chart eliminates the need to riffle through paper folders looking for information and replaces it with desktop mouse navigation that is much quicker and more productive. This last component is necessary to eliminate the paper chart and is important in realizing all of the benefits of electronic record keeping, because it can reduce significantly or eliminate the costs associated with storing and filing records. The surgeons need to enter data only into the EMR portion of the record documenting the doctor–patient visit. All other patient information is entered by clerical staff into the electronic chart by keyboard (demographics and billing) or scanning (eg, MRI and other reports). The three components of the electronic record need to be compatible but need not come from the same vender or company.

Advantages of the electronic medical record for the orthopedic surgeon

To make an EMR work for orthopedic surgeons, all the information they want to record about a patient must be available to them in an easily accessed program in a computer. These programs are derived from databases of set terms and concepts that describe historical, physical, laboratory, imaging, and therapeutic findings and actions. The terms correspond to every subjective complaint, physical finding, test result, and treatment modality employed by one or all specialties in medicine. These terms then are used to build a medical record by picking them individually or in groups in a pre-set fashion to populate the record with information. The terms must be standard enough to be recognized universally by clinicians but flexible and versatile enough to accommodate the variations in individual patients and physician practices.

The EMR should facilitate interaction with patients and speed office workflow by making it easier to produce and store patient information. An EMR should make the retrieval of past visits, diagnostic tests, therapeutic maneuvers, and surgical images much more efficient than storing this information in a paper chart. It should simplify intraoffice communication with an e-mail system and facilitate communication with other providers with on-line ordering of tests, therapies, and medicines. Back-office functions, such as filing and pulling charts, are eliminated, decreasing personnel costs. By automating many aspects of the documentation and ordering processes, an EMR theoretically will decrease the time it takes to see patients, allowing increased patient through-put in the office setting. These are the aspects of EMR that the RAND scientists envision when estimating all of those saved billions of dollars.

The theoretical advantages of an integrated EMR to an orthopedic practice are decreased operating costs, elimination of the costs associated with a paper chart, increased compliance in E&M documentation, automated Current Procedural Terminology (CPT) coding, centralized patient information, real-time generation of clinical notes, and the ability to access and analyze the clinical data generated by surgeons.

Transcription costs have become a significant budget line item for many practices. Currently, the going rate for transcription can be from 11 to 15 cents per line. This cost can be decreased by about half by outsourcing the transcription overseas; however, transcription still remains a significant operating cost. Add to this $3 to $6 in paper raw materials per patient plus the costs of filing, microfilming, and storage, and the potential savings produced by using an EMR become apparent [10].

Even with the most efficient dictation services there can be considerable delay in the time it takes to get a copy of a patient encounter into the chart. Patient care and safety are compromised when a dictation is not available. This problem can be especially common in larger practices in which a patient may be seen by multiple surgeons or at multiple sites. With an EMR, medical records are available instantaneously system wide. All the patient data for a given practice can be housed in a central location, permitting instant access from multiple sites. Practices that currently have more than one office location will benefit when treating the same patient at different sites. Data stored on a central server can be accessed securely from multiple sites by the Internet. Patient safety and satisfaction are increased with the constant availability of past medical history and treatment records. Decreasing redundancy and simplifying the retrieval of patient information enhances office efficiency. Surgeons can have access to patient records in the emergency room via hand held devices or at home and on the road via the Internet. This ready access facilitates care in night and weekend coverage situations and even can help track medication use and abuse.

The use of an EMR can increase compliance with current E&M coding principles with the proper use of templates. Although many practices use paper templates [5], the EMR has the benefit of automatically coding any given record. The EMR "counts the bullets" and determines the appropriate CPT code for the documentation provided. Many of the programs can prompt for deficiencies in documentation for coding for a given record. Electronic analysis ensures consistent proper coding.

Practices that do not conform to the coding guidelines run the risk of accusations of Medicare fraud. The government has the power to seize records for Medicare and Medicaid patients and to estimate the amount of "overcoding" based on the examination of a few records and then extrapolate this amount of overpayment to the practice's entire volume of these patients. This practice has not held up in court, but the time, expense, and bad publicity associated with such allegations are best avoided [11]. The managed care industry has seized on this method and begun retroactive claims denials against individual surgeons and practices. Managed Care Organizations (MCO) contracts usually stipulate the right of the MCO to review the medical records of their enrollees. The MCO reviews a sample of records for coding accuracy and then extrapolates alleged overcoding over the practice's entire covered population. The overcoding is alleged to be a breach of contract with the MCO and as such is governed by state contract law. In some states, such as New York, contract law states that monetary damage from breach of contract can be extrapolated over a 6-year period. The MCO then demands payment for alleged overpayments made for 6 years! Needless to say, this amount can add up quickly and usually not in favor of the surgeon. EMR is the perfect antidote to this situation. Because documentation of care has become the ultimate arbiter of physician reimbursement, it is essential that surgeons have a record system that accurately and consistently supports their level of coding. EMR, with the proper use of templates, does so in an automated fashion, increasing efficiency and providing insurance against claims of E&M coding errors. Compliance with the E&M coding guidelines has increased dramatically in the author's office with the use of the EMR.

The financial benefits of using an EMR averaged $33,000 per physician user per year in a recent study of family practice groups [6]. Financial benefits were obtained from two main sources: increased coding levels and efficiency-related savings or revenue gains. Each source contributed about 50% of the benefits. The efficiency-related gains were realized in decreased personnel and transcription costs and increased patient visits. Noticeably absent was any pay-for-performance reward from health insurers or Medicare. Each group realized enough gains to pay for the initial and cumulative EMR costs an average of 2.5 years after implementation and saw ongoing yearly net benefits of $23,000 per provider.

Savings in transcription costs have been the main benefit from using an EMR in the author's office. Before implementing the program, yearly transcription costs averaged $110,000 per year (Fig. 1). Current costs are $11,000 per year, and the majority of this cost is borne by the only surgeon still using dictation for record keeping. In addition, the equivalent of one full-time filing position has been eliminated, for a savings of $28,000 per year. The filing position was not eliminated until the author's group incorporated the program that allowed it to go to a paperless office. The group no longer purchases paper goods for charts, nor does it need to microfiche old records. The office area designated for chart storage is being converted into an additional examination room and will become an income-producing space for the practice. Savings from transcription alone paid for the cost of the project in 4 years with ongoing yearly savings of $87,000 per year ($99,000 savings in transcription plus $28,000 in personnel savings, minus $40,000 additional computer costs from EMR). This saving, which amounts to about $15,000 per surgeon per year, does not take into account decreased paper supply costs or any added benefit experienced from more accurate coding and billing.

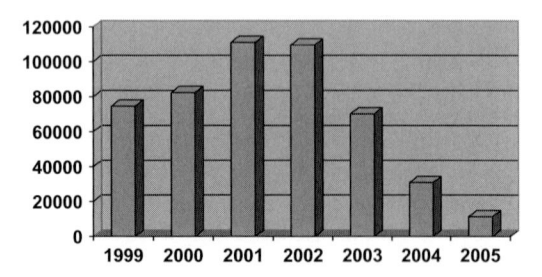

Fig. 1. Yearly transcription costs. EMR was implemented in April 2003.

Disadvantages of an electronic medical record

The disadvantages of an EMR are startup costs, difficulties in implementation, and impact on office workflow.

The monetary startup costs for an EMR system can be significant. The main costs associated with purchasing a system involve computer hardware, software, training, and service. These costs will vary widely depending on the specific system that is purchased. Systems can be purchased outright, purchased on an access-only basis, or leased. There can be licensing fees on a per-user basis. A comparison of these costs, as well as other attributes of EMR systems currently available, is accessible on the Internet at www.elmr-electronic-medical-records-emr.com [12].

Miller and colleagues [6] assessed the cost of adopting an EMR for solo practitioners and small groups of medical doctors and found that the average cost of implementing the record was $44,000 per physician with ongoing yearly costs of $8500 for each doctor. Table 1 lists all the costs the author's group incurred in the purchase of an EMR in 2001. The addition of an electronic chart and scanning program with scanning hardware in 2005 cost $50,000, for a total costs of $256,731, or $45,844 per surgeon. The group chose to finance this purchase over 5 years and incurred additional interest costs of $92,000 for a final total cost of $348,731, or $62,273 per surgeon. The group's ongoing yearly computer costs were $5000 per doctor without the EMR and increased to $12,000 per doctor with the EMR.

The use of EMR changes the routine with which doctors have become comfortable in their practice. Adoption of an EMR requires a considerable investment in physician time to learn the computer system and its applications. The less familiar a physician is with computer technology, the greater is the change in routine and the amount of time needed to learn the systems. Surgeons usually are fearful that adopting an EMR will slow office workflow and decrease income. Another worry is that the computerized record will not reflect the patient encounter accurately and that the user of the system and his colleagues will be unable to recognize the information that the EMR provides.

The learning curve in adopting the system will affect workflow for some amount of time. Surgeons differ in how they adopt the system. Some may choose to select certain types of encounters, such as postoperative visits or telephone calls, to practice entering data. Others may force themselves to use the programs full time. Some will adopt the systems easily, and some may not even want to try. Incentives, such as having those that do not adopt computerized records pay for their own transcription costs, can maximize use of an EMR. Making the decision to go to an EMR is one issue; getting doctors to use it is another! Once surgeons see the benefits of the system, it becomes easier to convince them to use it. Early adopters, therefore, have the responsibility to encourage use by demonstrating the advantages of EMR to their colleagues.

Miller [6] found that doctors worked longer hours for an average of 4 months following implementation of an EMR. This added work burden was not shared equally; physician "champions" of the EMR spent the most additional hours trying to integrate their systems. After an average 26 months of use, 11 of the 14 groups studied had "tightly integrated" the EMR into their practices, and 10 had gone to a completely paperless office. The author's office purchased the EMR in late 2001 but did not integrate the program fully until early in 2003. Two surgeons adopted the record early, and two more lagged by only a few months. Two additional surgeons never adopted the EMR but were able to adopt the electronic chart component, enabling the office to go completely paperless in 2005 when the group added an electronic chart. The champion surgeons spent more than 100 hours over a 5-month period developing the system for general use. It took 5 years from the time the group first contemplated an EMR until all of the benefits were realized.

Implementing an electronic medical record

The greatest challenge in implementing the EMR is the physical entry of clinical information by the surgeon into the computer. The process of entry must not affect office workflow adversely but must allow enough data to be collected for efficient analysis and retrieval. The problem is finding a format that allows the practitioner to enter data into the computer quickly and simply. The record should be generated in less time than it takes to dictate a standard office visit. The preparation of a quick and simple format is the most time-consuming aspect of implementing an EMR. It also is the essential for widespread use of the system in any given practice.

Table 1
Cost of electronic medical records and electronic charts

Item	Cost ($)
Workstations	18,000
Cruise pads	33,000
Server	4500
Laser printer	2600
Laser forms generator	1900
Printers	1250
Wireless local area network	4400
Electronic medical record software	81,200
Medical manager upgrade	8000
Instillation	16,000
Training	21,875
Support	14,000
Total	206,725
Lease interest	92,909.66
Total cost	299,634.66

Physicians have tried many different ways to enter data, including scanning paper documents, free text keyboard entry, voice recognition software, dictation, point-and-click entry, or combinations of these methods. Most of the systems on the market today employ a point-and-click method of data entry in a Windows or Windows-like graphic format. The point-and-click method seems to afford the most benefits in data entry, retrieval, and analysis. This format can be augmented with scanning, voice recognition, and keyboard entry to enhance the versatility of the system. Augmenting the system with these modalities allows a more individualized and descriptive record. The system, however, should capture as much data as possible using the point-and click method to avoid the need to modify the record with voice recognition or free text entry, because these methods currently are relatively inaccurate (voice) and time consuming (free text). Also, data added to the system in this manner usually are not recognized by the computer and therefore cannot be tracked or retrieved for future data analysis, negating one of the greatest advantages of computerized records.

The easiest way to assemble the EMR graphically is in template forms displayed on the computer terminal. Without these forms, too much time is needed to cull from a database all the necessary information to generate a note. If generating a note takes too much time or is awkward, surgeons will not adopt an EMR. Getting the information in the computer quickly and saved permanently and instantaneously ensures the successful implementation of an EMR. To speed information entry, systems must minimize the number of "clicks" needed to populate a record. The design and functionality of the templates dictates the speed of the record. In the author's office, the surgeons who spent the most time developing and refining their templates were the most satisfied with using the EMR.

The templates are best organized according to musculoskeletal areas and should be comprehensive. The screens displaying the information need to be easy to read and uncrowded. Therefore several screens usually are required to display all the data points. The user must be able to toggle through these screens instantaneously to populate the record with all the pertinent data. Separate screens for history, review of systems, physical examination, tests, diagnosis, and treatment help organize templates and make them more intuitive. Each screen should fit within a typical monitor screen so that data points always are in the same place. When the points are in the same place, the user's motor memory speeds data entry.

The EMR program can speed the templates with certain attributes. "Auto negative" buttons are very useful, because most historical and physical findings are negative. These buttons decrease the number of clicks necessary to enter information by automatically striking all the data points on a screen as negative. Pull-down lists for common adjectives and modifiers are needed to help increase the accuracy and completeness of the record. Free text boxes lend the ultimate ability to individualize a record but do require keyboard or voice activation entry, decreasing speed. Search functions are helpful in finding items in the database not included in the templates. The most effective function is the ability to save prepopulated templates that can be produced with one click. These templates can be generated for specific problems such as "Right Ankle Sprain" and are amended quickly and accurately for individual patients. This technique is especially powerful when dealing with routine office functions, such as postoperative visits, and conditions that present similarly across a population, such as lateral epicondylitis. Templates speed workflow dramatically and are quicker than standard dictation.

Production of templates is extremely time consuming, and most orthopedists will be unwilling to devote the time needed to develop them. It therefore is essential to have a library of orthopedic-specific templates available with the purchase of an EMR system. The templates need to satisfy all the previously discussed medical, legal, and economic functions to add value to the EMR. If the templates do not serve all three functions, the full value of the EMR will not be realized. Templates will allow a practice to "hit the ground running" with a system without the added start-up time for development. Many surgeons will complain that the templates do not reflect their current routines and therefore are inadequate for their needs. Unless they are willing to devote the time to develop their own templates or to modify existing ones slightly, they will have to alter their recordkeeping routines somewhat while adopting an EMR. The EMR should allow the addition and modification of templates, because as practitioners become more familiar with their systems, they will feel more comfortable and will want to have their own library of forms. As the EMR industry matures and more templates become available, this issue will become less important. For those who currently are deciding about the purchase of an EMR, however, having a system that provides a complete library of quality orthopedic templates is of primary importance.

The physical act of entering the data into the computer with a point-and-click method can be accomplished in several ways. The data can be entered in an office, examination room, or hallway workstation on a personal computer (PC) with a mouse or on a portable cruise pad or handheld device using a touch screen. Data entry to a PC is similar to other computer functions that many surgeons already perform and is attractive because of its familiarity. Physical access to data entry is limited unless multiple PCs are employed, but having PCs available at multiple sites increases hardware and licensing costs. The portable devices have the advantage of convenience of access but are hampered by limitations of battery life and speed. They require the use of wireless networks that can increase the amount of time needed to enter and save data. There are security concerns with wireless networks. The size of the viewing screens also is an issue: smaller screens are harder to see and make data entry more difficult. Portable tablets are currently available that have large, rotating liquid crystal display screens that solve the problem of screen size. These tablets are more expensive than PCs and also, unfortunately, are liable to theft.

The author's practice has tried data entry on PCs in doctor's offices, PCs at hallway workstations between examination rooms, wireless cruise pads, and wireless tablets. Mobile cruise pads with a wireless local area network proved to be inefficient because of the time required to enter data. Also, using the device in the presence of the patient is awkward, because the surgeon seems more interested in the cruise pad than in the patient's complaint! As a result, the $37,000 the author's group spent on portable cruise pads and a wireless network was an unnecessary expense.

The fastest and most consistent method of data entry seems to be PCs at workstations between examination rooms (Fig. 2). This set-up enhances workflow because the physician can enter data between seeing patients, while waiting for radiographs, and after injections . The author's group has tried augmenting the EMR with voice recognition software but has abandoned this technique in favor of keyboard entry. The reason is time: the corrections required while using voice recognition

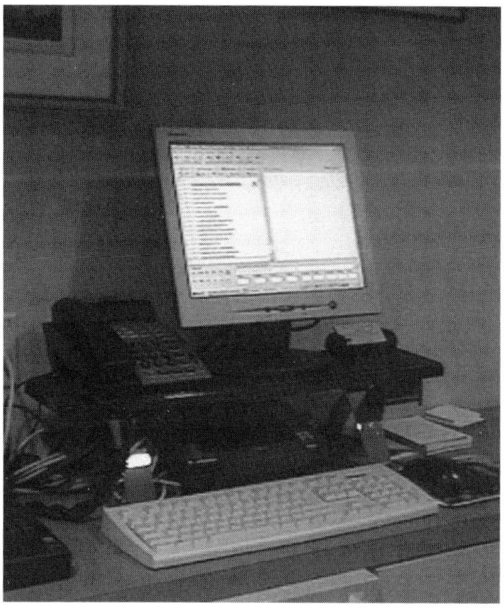

Fig. 2. Office workstation.

negate the time saved as compared with keystroke entry. With PC entry between workstations and a library of orthopedic templates, the author's group was able to implement the EMR system without significant impact on office workflow.

All paper correspondences that come into the office must be placed in the electronic chart. This entry is easy to accomplish by scanning the documents into the chart program to folders designated for various categories of information. Once the record is adopted, it is simple to start building new electronic charts with scanning and use of the EMR by the surgeons. The old paper charts, however, pose a challenge, in that all of their contents need to be scanned into the electronic chart to be available to the doctors and staff. Doing so takes considerable time and manpower. How a practice handles this problem will depend on the number of charts it has and how many are active. Higher percentages of active charts will require more aggressive scanning routines. The author's group began scanning charts based on the office schedule in 2-week blocks in April 2005. The old charts for all the patients scheduled during each 2 weeks were scanned into the program, and the charts of any additional unscheduled patients were scanned the evening before their visit. The group started with approximately 11,200 charts and has scanned 30% of them after 8 months of this scanning routine. Although this schedule is slower than scanning all the charts at once, it has allowed the group to get rid of the old charts gradually without hiring additional workers and even has permitted the group to eliminate a filing clerk position without undue burden on the rest of the staff.

Recommendations for considering an electronic medical record

At this point the decision to adopt an EMR is primarily a business decision and as such should be made with both costs and benefits in mind. A practice must understand all the costs of its paper chart and compare that with the cost of an EMR. The decision to purchase an EMR will make sense when an analysis of the return on investment is agreed to be favorable for a given practice. There are other ways to decrease transcription costs and comply with regulations, such as the use of paper templated systems [5,13], which are far less costly and disruptive than the use of an EMR. These options should be considered when deciding to purchase an EMR. The costs can be significant, and the financial benefits usually are not realized until a few years after adoption. Ongoing savings, however, can be substantial and should be considered a primary goal when investing in an EMR.

There should be consensus among the members of a practice to purchase an EMR, because implementation is difficult even for those who are committed. It took 19 months to integrate the EMR in the author's practice because of simple inertia, even though the group was committed to and was paying for the EMR! The process of building consensus takes time. One or two members of the group who are familiar with computer systems should be appointed to research the project. They will need to compare several systems before one can be chosen. It is best to start with a system that is available through or that interfaces with the electronic billing system that a practice currently uses. They then should explore systems that other physicians in the area are using. It is better to examine those that are used specifically by other orthopedic surgeons to ensure that the program fulfills the specific needs of the specialty. It is helpful to visit sites where the systems are in use to get a good sense of how they function in the clinical setting. Questions concerning the reliability of the program and its support should be directed to both the doctors using the system and to the administrative staff for a comprehensive evaluation of the program.

The stability of the company marketing the EMR and the vendor servicing it should be investigated. Because of the dynamism of the current marketplace, companies form, merge, and fail with alarming frequency. The author's group purchased its EMR from a vendor that lost the ability to service the program because of changes in the corporate structure and policies of the company that developed the program. This development significantly complicated the adoption of the program.

The future

The widespread use of electronic records and their storage in Regional Health Information Organizations is a goal of many health care policy experts [14]. They view the adoption of such a national system as a necessity in controlling health care spending, managing disease states, identifying the occurrence of disease, and protecting homeland security. Not all experts agree with the assessment that EMR will provide the myriad of benefits that are proposed, and some contend that the current enthusiasm is unwarranted and based on unproven assumptions [7]. There is, however, great interest in the public sector in EMR and in encouraging physicians to migrate toward electronic record keeping [1–3,14]. Further complicating the discussion is that the different stakeholders in the system have competing interests regarding the use of EMR. Although all may want "improved quality," Medicare and insurers are interested primarily in cutting overall spending. Providers may not benefit from such a decrease in spending and will have to be compensated in some fashion for using EMR. Conversely, providers currently using EMR actually may increase spending by improving their reimbursement with better coding compliance, to the detriment of the third-party payers! Despite all the enthusiasm about the potential of EMR, however, it does not seem that there will be a mandate to use it, or to pay for it, in the near future.

Currently, EMR makes sense for orthopedic surgeons only if they determine that it is a sound business decision. In the future, the electronic analysis of treatment outcomes that EMR affords may be attractive to orthopedic surgeons and other providers. EMR will allow examination of practice patterns in regards to both cost and effectiveness. Individual surgeons and practices will be able to track treatment protocols and results without the high cost in time and manpower currently needed to collect and analyze such information. This type of information is going to be of great value to both patients and surgeons in the quest to evaluate and provide quality health care. Currently, there is no way for patients, those who purchase health care (businesses), or doctors to assess the true value of what they are buying or providing. There has been an explosion of companies that try to provide this type of information, but the development of this industry has been hampered by the difficulty in obtaining quality information from "messy folders stuffed with hand-scribbled notes" [15]. Widespread use of EMR will make these data easier to obtain and will lead to some type of standard system to evaluate "quality." Orthopedics lends itself well to this type of evaluation because of the definitive treatment endpoints of reduction of pain and improvement of function that musculoskeletal medicine possesses. With this information, it will be possible to demonstrate the value of orthopedic care. When value is demonstrated, the ever-downward spiral of physician reimbursement will end, because price no longer will be the only means to compare different health plans and providers, and quality of care will be the more important determinant. Surgeons who supply this quality care will be in great demand, and those in demand will command appropriate reimbursement [4]. The recent trend of shifting costs back to patients with increased deductibles and copayments plus the provision for Health Savings Accounts in the last Medicare reform package may hasten the demand for information regarding quality of services.

EMR is an emerging technology that will impact the practice of medicine in the coming years. Several powerful trends are making the transition to an electronic record favorable; in the future it may be mandatory. By embracing and affecting this technology early, orthopedic surgeons will be in a position to make this transition work for them.

References

[1] Bower A. The diffusion and value of healthcare information technology. Pub. No. MG-272-HLTH. Santa Monica (CA): RAND Corporation; 2005.

[2] Hillestad R, Bigelow J, Bower A, et al. Can electronic medical record systems transform health care? Potential health benefits, savings and costs. Health Aff 2005;24:1103–17.

[3] Tang P. Key capabilities of an electronic health record system. Committee on data standards for patient safety. Board on Health Care Services. Institute of Medicine. Washington, DC: The National Academy Press; 2003.

[4] McIntyre L. Making the electronic medical record work for the orthopedic surgeon. Sports Med Arthrosc 2004;12:238–45.

[5] ORTHOcoderMD. Available at: http://www.orthocoder.com. Accessed February 10, 2004.

[6] Miller R, West C, Brown TM, et al. The value of electronic health records in solo or small group practices. Health Aff 2005;24:1127–37 2005.

[7] Himmelstein D, Woolhandler S. Hope and hype: predicting the impact of electronic medical records. Health Aff 2005;24:1121–3.

[8] Physician socioeconomic statistics. 2002–2003 edition. Chicago: American Medical Association; 2002.

[9] American Medical Association. Current procedural terminology. 5th edition. Chicago: American Medical Association; 2003.

[10] Soper WD. Why I love my EMR. Fam Pract Manag 2002;9(9):35–8.

[11] Hawryluk M. CMS initiative cuts doctor-despised Medicare audit procedure. Available at: http://www.ama-assn.org/amednews/2002/06/17/gvsa0617.htm. Accessed November 19, 2003.

[12] Voelker KG. Electronic medical record (EMR) comparison by physicians for physicians. Available at: http://www.elmr-electronic-medical-records-emr.com. Accessed January 21, 2004.

[13] Beach WR, Ritchie J, Bert JM. Coding and reimbursement in arthroscopic surgery. Arthroscopy 2002;18(Suppl 1):96–121.

[14] Center for Health Transformation. Accelerating transformation through health information technology. Available at: http://www.healthtransformation.net/cs/news/news_detail?pressrelease.id=591. Accessed November 15, 2007.

[15] Herzlinger R. Market driven health care: who wins, who loses in the transformation of America's largest service industry. Reading (MA): Addison-Wesley; 1997.

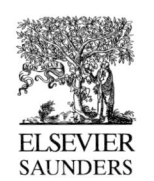

Putting It All Together: The Efficient, Profitable Orthopedic Practice

Jack M. Bert, MD

Summit Orthopedics, Ltd., 17 W. Exchange Street, Suite 307, St. Paul, MN 55102, USA

In today's complex practice environment, the orthopedic surgeon is faced with multiple stressful practice decisions. To achieve a surgeon's personal practice goals of quality of care, quality of life, and improvement in quality of practice, the physician must commit himself or herself to a certain amount of restructuring of his or her practice. Part of this reorganization should involve bringing "in house" as many ancillary services as the practice can support. Doing so will create efficiencies both in the clinic and in surgical practice. Furthermore, an the orthopedist who is able to improve his or her personal effectiveness and efficiency in the clinic and the operating room will achieve a tremendous level of satisfaction as a result.

Creating a high quality of care within the practice setting requires the ability to refer for appropriate tests and administer necessary treatment without concern for the expenses incurred. This quality of care can be achieved by having the physician group control its own ancillary services that allow the orthopedist to schedule these services immediately and control costs as necessary but still negotiate contractual agreements with the payers.

Quality of life relates to the orthopedist's ability to regain some control of the practice environment. Owning, managing, and controlling ancillary services, even if there is a joint venture agreement, gives the group the greatest ability to control patient care and revenue. Furthermore, creating a large, diverse group of orthopedic surgeons covering extensive geography in the local marketplace allows the group to negotiate with insurers and hospital systems from a position of strength. Improvements in office and operating room efficiencies will allow the orthopedist to work more effectively and with greater enjoyment.

Quality of practice, therefore, is a combination of quality of care, quality of life, and, in addition, quality of income. Quality of income relates to appropriate reimbursement for work generated. As the costs of goods and services continue to increase, as the consumer price index rises, and as reimbursements continue to decline, a dramatic increase in group overhead usually results. The orthopedic group must strive to achieve the best payer mix possible and, if necessary, must renegotiate or eliminate poor-paying contracts, especially those with withholds. Doing so is especially difficult if the orthopedic group is small and the environment in the group's marketplace is highly competitive.

A surgeon's personal efficiency and expediency in both the operating room and clinic can be self-taught with the proper attitude. The advantages of working efficiently in the operating room include improved outcomes, economic rewards, and time savings. As stated by Rob Booth, MD, from University of Pennsylvania, who is a very fast surgeon, "Be quick in the operating room, but don't hurry. Concentrate on being effective and efficient, not necessarily on being fast as that will follow naturally. We can all improve!" (R. Booth, MD, personal communication, 2001). Maurice Mueller, MD, once stated, "The operating room is a bad place to think" (M. Mueller, MD, personal communication, 1985). He meant that orthopedists should standardize procedures so that they are performing perhaps only 20 to 30 steps in an operation, rather than varying the surgical technique intraoperatively and continually trying

E-mail address: bertx001@tc.umn.edu

to "figure it out as they go." A former partner of the author's continually reminded the scrub nurse when she did not hand him the correct instrument, "I do it the same way every time!" (C. Tountas, MD, personal communication) This orthopedist was a very efficient and speedy surgeon, and his message was clear. If the surgeon can learn to operate efficiently, reproducibly, with ability and expertise, it will make the orthopedist's workday more enjoyable and a lot easier than arriving late to a clinic full of upset patients.

Fred Taylor, who died at the age of 50 in 1915, developed the assembly line manufacturing process that is still in use today. His theory was that "to improve the performance of a machine, you had to improve the performance of the workers that ran the machine" (F. Taylor, personal communication, 1987). To obtain a truly high-quality, efficient practice, the orthopedist must improve his or her own performance and the performance of those associated with the care delivery team. Unfortunately, doing so involves a willingness to change habits, which can be very difficult. For those willing to consider change, however, office efficiencies can be developed that involve restructuring the clinic setting and staffing it with the best team of employees available who share the orthopedist's goals. This commitment to providing high-quality care begins at the front desk, the entry point for the patient. Optimally, the history intake form has been sent to the patient and filled out in advance. Otherwise, a friendly, courteous front-desk person must be willing to help the patient fill out the form if necessary. An unhelpful, discourteous receptionist can create a negative experience for patients within the clinic setting. Ideally, the office examination area itself consists of modules of four rooms with a secretarial space across from this group of rooms. This arrangement allows the secretary to be in close contact with the orthopedist and the physician assistant (PA) at all times. The secretary and PA are necessary members of the clinical team and are critical to obtaining maximum office efficiency. The secretary manages the clinic and schedules MRI scans, consultations, surgical procedures, physical therapy appointments, and return appointments if she has time. She must precertify all surgical procedures. All incoming physician calls must be screened by the clinical team; first by the secretary and then by the PA, before they are ever diverted to the orthopedist. The x-ray technician, front-desk person, and/or the secretary rooms patients and does whatever is necessary to improve patient flow. The PA or medical assistant should assist in rooming patients and performing suture removal, dressing changes, casting, and joint injections. The PA schedules MRIs and consultations, as necessary, when the secretary is busy with another patient. The PA also must be committed to do whatever is necessary to improve patient flow. A critical aspect of the PA's responsibilities during clinics is to answer questions regarding injury care, surgery, and patient concerns after the orthopedist leaves the room. The primary goal of the clinical care team is to answer all patient questions satisfactorily and then manage the patient properly after the physician completes his or her contact with the patient. The clinical care team must complete certification and scheduling of any further testing, surgery, or consultation before the patient leaves the office unless the secretary makes arrangements for the patient to contact them later after the clinic is completed.

Within the orthopedic clinic setting, the patient care team is absolutely critical. The orthopedist must delegate responsibility to others to avoid being bogged down with insignificant tasks that can be handled easily by ancillary personnel. The key to success for physician efficiency therefore is to delegate responsibility. Some physicians find delegating very difficult because they are afraid to allow others to perform clinical responsibilities that they perceive as difficult or that are potentially at risk for complications. When the physician has successfully trained his staff to perform routine care and treatment, he or she must be willing to allow the staff to work without continued micromanagement. Otherwise, this system will fail, become extremely inefficient, and become frustrating for both the staff and the orthopedist. Furthermore, it will result in poor staff morale because the staff will detect the orthopedist's unwillingness to trust them to do their work. The willingness to delegate is the primary reason some physicians are efficient and the majority of physicians are not. If the physician can delegate responsibility and has a high-quality staff, he or she should be able to involve the clinical care team in the care of the patient as soon as the diagnosis is made and treatment has been offered.

It is the surgeon's job to train the clinical team to work in the clinic the way that he or she wants them to. Just like the workers on the assembly machine, they must improve their performance to provide an efficient, high-quality clinical service. As their "teacher," the surgeon must treat his employees with respect; otherwise, the care team will not perform for the physician, and any efficiency that might be gained will be lost. During the patient care process, it is important to remember that the physician should be doing the work that he or she was trained to do and should let the clinical care team take care of the noncritical tasks of patient care. The orthopedist should orchestrate his clinic by delegating as much as authority as possible to his clinical team and should focus on working through the clinic quickly and efficiently while still doing as good a job with the patients as possible. The time spent with each patient is termed "physician encounter time," and the time his clinical team spends with each patient is termed "team encounter time." The goal of the orthopedist is to reduce physician encounter time and increase the team encounter time while providing high-quality patient care. If this goal can be achieved, the orthopedist will have more time to see a larger number of patients and will answer only critical clinical questions that his team feels uncomfortable answering.

An example of this sequence is a new patient consult entering the office for the first visit. The history form for a level 5 examination should be completed by the patient if it has not already been completed before the visit. The PA then reviews the history form, fills out a joint examination template for a level 3 examination, if applicable, organizes any pre-existing medical record, and obtains the necessary radiographs. The orthopedist then evaluates the patient after reviewing the medical history form and examination template and manages the patient. If the treatment is conservative, the PA can write and sign prescriptions and work restrictions under the orthopedist's direction. If the treatment is surgical, the PA can review the surgical procedure and its potential complications with the patient. The PA then directs the patient to the secretary for scheduling of consultations, tests, or further surgery with completion of certification. In the meantime, the PA is working up a new patient, changing a cast, or removing sutures, and the secretary is helping to manage the patient. If the patient has any other clinical questions, the PA is ready to answer them after he or she has completed other clinical tasks. Surgeons who use their care team in this fashion always seem to be the largest producers in virtually any orthopedic group practice.

If delegation is the heart of time management, then focus is the soul of time management. The orthopedist should concentrate on each patient and get right to the problem immediately. He or she should diagnose the condition rapidly, offer treatment and further testing, and then let the clinical team take over care of the patient. This sequence is the key to an efficient clinical office practice.

Most orthopedic surgeons work long hours and work hard, but very few work "smart." Smart physicians abolish downtime, but decreasing downtime requires both an efficient support team and accessible ancillary services. Delegating and focusing on the office clinic work and adding ancillary services wherever possible will allow the orthopedist to improve efficiency and profitability dramatically. It is important to never travel to more than one location during the day. One always should schedule surgeries at the hospital or ASC closest to the clinic where the orthopedist is currently working. Traveling by car to another location adds an additional hour of time to the surgeon's day. The results are always surprising to the physician when this "windshield time" or downtime over the course of a week is added up. When one counts every minute from the time the surgeon leaves one location, goes to the preoperative area, waits for the patient to be brought into the operating room, completes the case, writes orders, discusses the case with the relatives, and travels again to a different location to perform another surgery, the amount of time is always significant. Once the orthopedic group has its own ancillary services or a joint venture with a hospital or other group, appropriate scheduling should be mandatory to help abolish the downtime associated with traveling to multiple locations. If the group becomes large enough, partners can share in call rounding responsibilities at different hospital locations.

Increasing group size is critical to obtain increased throughput of ancillary services, to negotiate payer contracts from a position of strength, to increase market share by offering multiple clinic locations, to reduce the frequency of call responsibilities, and to improve fraternity within the group as a dominating presence in the community. Very few payers care about a small orthopedic group unless there is no other choice in the community, because payers want geographic coverage to provide convenience for its plan members. Size does not necessarily guarantee profitability and success, but it will guarantee inclusion in most managed care contract negotiations. If the group is unwilling to do a full-asset merger with additional orthopedic groups in its marketplace because of personal or cultural issues, an umbrella merger may make sense to see if the mix of cultures and new partners is tolerable. By combining groups in this way, separate divisions are maintained, but the umbrella corporation bills for the divisions with a single provider number. The umbrella corporation is the contracting entity and is comprised of board members from each group, but each division is managed locally. The benefits of an umbrella corporation are that it avoids the "bigness" within each division; it is a single contracting entity; it allows for wider catchment area; and the mergers are much easier. If the merger works, the new entity will have increased dramatically its clout in the marketplace and influence on the payers. It furthermore improves the group's ability to make ancillary services tremendously profitable through increased patient volumes offsetting fixed overhead expense.

The efficient, profitable orthopedic practice must have strong, aggressive management. It must attempt to obtain the highest reimbursement possible by negotiating favorable rates with all insurers and health maintenance organizations from a position of strength that can be achieved only by becoming bigger. The practice should strive to have the best possible payer mix by eliminating poor-paying contracts. It should attempt to develop practice efficiencies by controlling as many ancillary services as possible and to provide high-quality care by choosing the best employees possible to administer those ancillary services. The group must employ a high-quality care team that will provide excellent patient care services under each orthopedist's direction. The author believes that quality of care is improved significantly by bringing ancillary services under physician control. The orthopedist can choose who delivers the care—the nurses employed in the ambulatory surgery center, the radiologist who reads the MRI scan performed at the group's scanner, and the physical therapist who administers the rehabilitative therapy. These in-house services allow greater control over the quality of the services rendered and allow management of the costs of that service

Finally, rigid personalities that are unwilling to change have no chance of adapting to the constantly changing health care delivery environment. Rigidity is not confined to age. The author has witnessed older partners being willing to learn new techniques and being open minded about more modern treatments, whereas some younger partners actually have said, "I'm getting too old to change." Change will continue to happen in the medical care industry, and the successful orthopedic group must adjust and adapt to it as quickly as possible. Positive change should be enjoyable and should not be feared. Physicians who are willing to be flexible will succeed with change, but those who are rigid and inflexible will not. Rigidity arises from insecurity of the unknown; it is an unwillingness to be creative and try to step "out of the box" to learn a technique or business strategy that may be challenging and difficult to adapt to. It also is important to be unwilling to quit if a technique is difficult to learn. To be rigid is academically stifling and in the author's opinion is the hallmark trait of a mediocre physician, regardless of specialty.

The orthopedist who is willing to be flexible, who works to put in the time and effort to become more efficient and effective, and who strives continuously to be an excellent surgeon and clinician will find that work becomes both more enjoyable and more profitable. Furthermore, by attempting to control the orthopedic marketplace by merging groups and increasing the size of the group, the orthopedist ultimately will have greater control over the quality of the patient's medical care.

Further reading

JM Bert. Guest Editor Practice management. Clin Sports Med 2002;21(2):321–5.

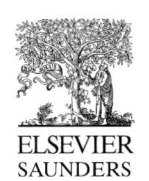

Index

Note: Page numbers of article titles are in **boldface** type.

A

Ambulatory surgery center(s)
  development of, **17–25**
    construction of, 22–23
    design in, 22
    equipment for, 23
    feasibility analysis in, 19–20
    legal issues in, 20
    licensure and certification in, 23–24
    partnership/ownership options in, 20–21
    policies related to, 23
    procedures in, 23
    reasons for, 17
    regulatory issues in, 20
    site location in, 21–22
    steps in, 19–24
  federal and state level attacks on, 109
  future prospects for, 25
  management of, 24–25
  single-specialty advantages of, 17–18
  specialty hospitals vs., 18–19
  within group practice, analysis of, 97

Ambulatory surgery center joint ventures
  cons of, 14–15
  pros of, **11–14**
    access to legal council, 14
    developing patient referral patterns, 11–12
    payer contracts, 13–14
    physical owner as manager, 12–13
    potential for protection against legislation restricting practice and development, 12
    shared investment and risk, 13
    supply and services contracting, 13
    training and education, 14

Ambulatory surgical center joint ventures, analysis of, 97–98

Ancillary service(s)
  available to orthopedic surgeon, **1–4**
    current climate, 1–2
    group size, 3–4
    independent medical examination companies, 3
    in-office durable medical equipment, 3
    in-office MRI units, 3
    in-office surgery center, 2–3
    occupational health services, 3
    physical therapy services, 3
  feasibility study related to, **5–9**
  legal issues affecting, **89–102**
    insurance contracts, 97
    investigations-related, 100–102
    Stark law, 92–97
    state law–related, 97
  market analysis related to, **5–9**
  opportunities for, analysis of, 97–100
    ambulatory surgical center joint ventures, 97–98
    ambulatory surgical centers within group practice, 97
    diagnostic test–related, 99–100
    occupational therapy services, 99
    physical therapy services, 99
    radiology services, 98–99
    referrals from unaffiliated physicians, 98

Ancillary service providers, at federal and state level
  attack on, **103–120**
    ambulatory surgery centers–related, 109
    balance of power–related, 113–114
    certificate of need, 109–110
    medical community–related, 108–109
    public relations
      against niche providers and organized medicine's fragmented response, 110–113
      American Hospital Association case studies on niche provider restrictions, 111–112
      Jean Mitchell, 2005 specialty hospital studies, 110–111
      Missouri Hospital Association, 112–113

Ancillary service providers (*continued*)
    specialty hospital regulatory environment, effect on transactional marketplace, 113
    threat from specialty and niche providers, 114
    Centers for Medicare and Medicaid Services' refusal to certify new specialty hospitals for Medicare reimbursement, 105
    history of, 113
    Medicare Payment Advisory Commission on extending moratorium, 108
    recent developments, 104–110
    research observations and findings related to, 115–116
    terminology related to, 113
    trends, 104–110, 113
    United States Congressional initiatives, 107–108
    United States Senate bill to reinstate moratorium, 106–107

Anti-kickback statute, of Medicare, 90–92

C

Centers for Medicare and Medicaid Services, refusal to certify new specialty hospitals for Medicare reimbursement, 105

Certificate of need, federal and state level attacks on, 109–110

Congress, 91

Contract(s), insurance, affecting ancillary services and orthopedic practice, 97

D

Diagnostic tests, supervision of and billing for, analysis of, 99–100

Drug testing, in physician-owned occupational health department, 65–67

Durable-medical equipment (DME) service, physician-owned, **71–79**
    creation of, 75–78
    described, 71
    enhancement of, 75–78
    obstacles related to, 78–79
    options for practice, 74–75
    practice assessment, 71–73

E

Electronic medical record (EMR), **121–129**
    advantages of, 123–124
    disadvantages of, 124–125
    future of, 128–129
    implementation of, 125–128
    recommendations for consideration of, 128
    structure and function of, 121–123

EMR. See *Electronic medical record (EMR)*.

F

Feasibility studies, ancillary services-related, **5–9**

G

Gain-sharing, with hospital
    continuing evolution related to, 36
    described, 35
    in current legal environment, **33–36**
        described, 33–34
        improvements in, 36
        navigating regulatory issues, 35–36
        "phynanical" relationships, 34–35

GAO. See *Government Accountability Oce (GAO)*.

Government Accountability Office (GAO), 105

H

Health care industry, in U.S., monies related to, 121

Health Insurance Portability and Accountability Act (HIPAA), 91

HIPAA. See *Health Insurance Portability and Accountability Act (HIPAA)*.

Hospital(s). See also specific types.
    specialty, ambulatory surgery center vs., 18–19

I

Imaging center(s)
    history of, from orthopedic perspective, 37
    physician-owned, **37–48**
        comparison with outside imaging, 42
        considerations in, 46
        economics of, 46–47
        financing for, 45–46
        MRI
            advent of, 37–42
            case example, 44–45
            evaluation of, 42–44

Independent medical examination(s) (IMEs)
    described, 81
    overview of, 81

Independent medical examination (IME) company
  available to orthopedic surgeon, 3
  physician-owned, **81–87**
    management style and shared vision, 85–86
    staff and skill sets, 86–87
    start-up considerations, 82–85
In-office durable medical equipment, available to orthopedic surgeon, 3
In-office MRI units, available to orthopedic surgeon, 3
In-office surgery center, available to orthopedic surgeon, 2–3
Insurance contracts, affecting ancillary services and orthopedic practice, 97

L

Law(s)
  Stark, 92–97
  state, affecting ancillary services and orthopedic practice, 97
Legal environment, in gain-sharing with hospital, **33–36**. See also *Gain-sharing, with hospital, in current legal environment.*
Legal issues
  ancillary-related, **89–102**
  in ambulatory surgery center development, 20
  orthopedic practice–related, **27–40**

M

Magnetic resonance imaging (MRI), advent of, 37–42
Market analysis, ancillary services–related, **5–9**
Medical group practice, financing and cash flow management for, **27–31**
  business plan, 27–30
    bank relationship, 29
    capital, 29
    capital call, 29–30
    equipment leasing and purchasing, 30
    financial plan, 28
    financing needs, 28
    non-recourse loans, 31
    practice description, 27–28
    pro-forma analysis, 28–29
  capital or financing lease, 30
  operating lease, 30
  recourse loans, 31
  terminology related to, 30–31

Medical record, structure and function of, 121–123
Medicare, 89–90
  anti-kickback statute of, 90–92
Missouri Hospital Association, attack on, 112–113
Mitchell, Jean, 2005 specialty hospital studies, 110–111
MRI. See *Magnetic resonance imaging (MRI).*

O

Occupational health department, physician-owned, **55–69**
  customer retention, 67
  drug testing in, 65–67
  financial considerations related to, 61
  marketing occupational medicine program, 59–61
  opportunities in, 61–65
  planning clinical operation, 57–59
  preliminary assessments in, 55–57
    competitory survey, 56
    employer market survey, 56
    location, 55
    profit margins, 56–57
    quantifying market potential, 55–56
    service issues, 56
Occupational health services, available to orthopedic surgeon, 3
Occupational medicine, opportunities in, in current environment, 61–65
  background of, 61
  described, 62–63
  experience modification ratings, 61–62
  quandaries, 62–63
Occupational medicine program, marketing of, 59–61
Occupational therapy services, analysis of, 99
Orthopedic practice, legal issues affecting, **89–102**
  insurance contracts, 97
  investigations-related, 100–102
  Stark law, 92–97
  state-law related, 97
Orthopedic surgeon
  ancillary services available to, **1–4**. See also *Ancillary service(s), available to orthopedic surgeon.*

making EMR work for. See also *Electronic medical record (EMR)*.

P

Partnership/ownership options, in ambulatory surgery center development, 20–21

Physical therapy department, physician-owned, **49–53**

Physical therapy services
analysis of, 99
available to orthopedic surgeon, 3

Physician-owned imaging centers, **37–48**. See also *Imaging center(s), physician-owned*.

Physician-owned IME company, **81–87**. See also *Independent medical examination (IME) company, physician-owned*.

Physician-owned occupational health department, **55–69**. See also *Occupational health department, physician-owned*.

Physician-owned physical therapy department, **49–53**

Portable orthopedic practice, **131–134**

Public relations, attacks at federal and state level, 110–113. See also *Ancillary service providers, at federal and state level, attack on, public relations*.

Q

Quality of advice, evaluation of, tips for, 89–90

R

Radiology services, analysis of, 98–99

RAND Corporation, 121

Referral(s), from unaffiliated physicians, analysis of, 98

Regulatory issues, in ambulatory surgery center development, 20

Ryan Associates, 56

S

Specialty hospital moratorium, June 2005 expiration of, 105–106

Specialty hospitals, ambulatory surgery center vs., 18–19

Stark law, 92–97

State laws, affecting ancillary services and orthopedic practice, 97

U

United States Congressional initiatives, 107–108

United States Senate bill to reinstate moratorium, 106–107

Moving?

Make sure your subscription moves with you!

To notify us of your new address, find your **Clinics Account Number** (located on your mailing label above your name), and contact customer service at:

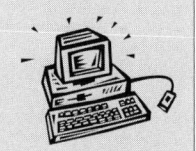

E-mail: elspcs@elsevier.com

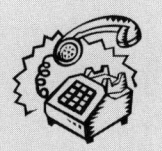

800-654-2452 (subscribers in the U.S. & Canada)
407-345-4000 (subscribers outside of the U.S. & Canada)

Fax number: 407-363-9661

Elsevier Periodicals Customer Service
6277 Sea Harbor Drive
Orlando, FL 32887-4800

*To ensure uninterrupted delivery of your subscription, please notify us at least 4 weeks in advance of move.

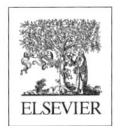

ELSEVIER